# Neck Pain Unveiled

A Comprehensive Guide to Understanding and Overcoming Neck Pain

Branko Weitzmann

**PUBLISHED BY: CKV Publishing,
Branko Weitzmann**

**ISBN: 978-1-4452-4420-4**

**Cover design: Tenisha Weitzmann
@ Instagram: teeniitravels**

**Disclaimer**
This book is intended to provide information and entertainment to the reader. The content presented in this book is the result of research and knowledge available as of the date of its publication, which is [publication date]. The author and the publishers have made every reasonable effort to ensure that the information contained in this book is accurate and up to date at the time of its printing.

However, because the information in this book is subject to constant change and evolution, it cannot be guaranteed to be completely free of errors or to reflect the most current information at the time of reading.

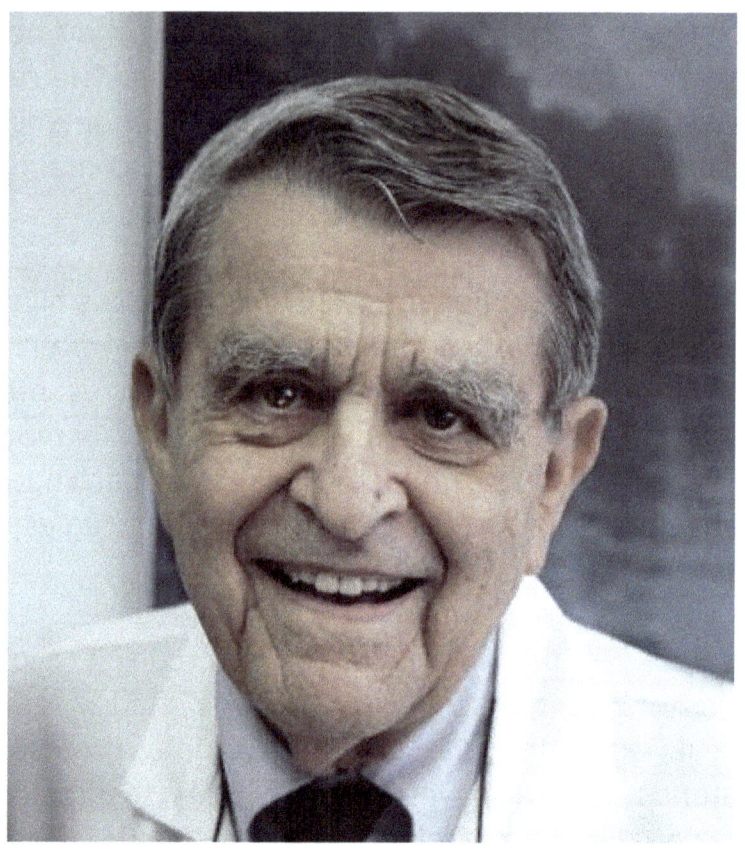

*"There is probably no other medical condition which is treated in so many different ways and by such a variety of practitioners as back pain. Though the conclusion may be uncomfortable, the medical community must bear the responsibility for this, for it has been distressingly narrow in its approach to the problem."*

– John Sarno

# Table of Contents

**Preface**

**Chapter 1: Understanding Neck Pain**
1. Anatomy of the neck
2. Common causes of neck pain
3. Types of neck pain (acute, chronic, etc.)

**Chapter 2: Diagnosis and Assessment**
1. Medical history and physical examination
2. Imaging and diagnostic tests
3. Assessing the impact on daily life and function

**Chapter 3: Non-Specific Neck Pain**
1. Exploring non-specific neck pain
2. Contributing factors and risk factors
3. Management and treatment options

**Chapter 4: Specific Neck Conditions**
1. Cervical spondylosis
2. Cervical radiculopathy
3. Whiplash-associated disorders and other specific
   conditions

**Chapter 5: Conservative Treatment Approaches**
1. Physical therapy and exercise
2. Pain management techniques
3. Lifestyle modifications and ergonomic considerations

## Chapter 6: Interventional and Surgical Options
1. Epidural steroid injections
2. Minimally invasive procedures
3. Surgical interventions for specific conditions

## Chapter 7: Complementary and Alternative Therapies
1. Acupuncture and acupressure
2. Chiropractic care
3. Mind-body approaches (yoga, meditation)

## Chapter 8: Psychological and Emotional Impact
1. Coping with chronic pain
2. Addressing psychological factors
3. Support for mental well-being

## Chapter 9: Preventing and Managing Recurrences
1. Strategies for preventing future episodes
2. Rehabilitation and long-term management
3. Red flags and when to seek medical attention

## Chapter 10: Living with Neck Pain
1. Maintaining quality of life
2. Support networks and resources
3. Advocacy and raising awareness

## Epilogue

## Acknowledgements

## Appendices
- Books

- Websites
- Organizations
- YouTube Channels
- Best Neck Stretches
- Best Strength Exercises for your Neck

## More interesting books by Branko Weitzmann

## References

# Preface

Neck pain is a common and often debilitating condition that affects millions of people worldwide. It can be caused by a variety of factors, including poor posture, muscle strain, injury, or underlying medical conditions. The impact of neck pain on an individual's quality of life can be significant, affecting their ability to work, engage in physical activities, and even perform simple daily tasks. As a result, finding effective ways to manage and alleviate neck pain is of paramount importance.

This book aims to provide a comprehensive and accessible resource for individuals suffering from neck pain, as well as for healthcare professionals seeking to expand their knowledge in this area. Drawing on the latest research and clinical expertise, we have compiled a wealth of information on the causes, symptoms, diagnosis, and treatment of neck pain. Our goal is to empower readers with the knowledge and tools they need to better understand their condition and make informed decisions about their care.

In the first section of this book, we delve into the anatomy and biomechanics of the neck, providing a foundational understanding of the structures involved and how they function. We explore common causes of neck pain, from everyday activities such as poor posture and prolonged sitting to more serious issues like whiplash injuries and degenerative conditions. By gaining insight into the underlying mechanisms of neck pain, readers can develop a clearer picture of why they may be experiencing discomfort and what steps they can take to address it.

The subsequent sections of the book focus on various aspects of managing and treating neck pain. We discuss conservative approaches such as exercise, physical therapy, and ergonomic modifications, as well as more advanced interventions including medications, injections, and surgical options. Additionally, we explore complementary and alternative therapies that may offer relief for some individuals. Throughout these discussions, we emphasize the importance of personalized care, recognizing that each person's experience with neck pain is unique and may require a tailored approach.

Furthermore, we address the psychological and emotional impact of chronic neck pain, acknowledging the toll it can take on mental well-being and overall quality of life. By integrating strategies for coping with the emotional aspects of pain, we aim to provide a holistic perspective on managing neck pain and promoting overall wellness.

It is important to note that this book is not a substitute for professional medical advice. Readers are encouraged to consult with qualified healthcare providers to receive personalized evaluations and recommendations tailored to their specific needs. Our intention is to complement, not replace, the guidance of healthcare professionals, and to serve as a valuable resource for enhancing the dialogue between patients and their care teams.

In compiling this book, we have drawn upon the expertise of leading healthcare professionals, researchers, and individuals with lived experience of neck pain. Their contributions have been invaluable in shaping the content and ensuring its relevance to those affected by this condition.

We hope that this book serves as a beacon of knowledge and empowerment for individuals grappling with neck pain, as well as a source of inspiration and guidance for healthcare professionals dedicated to improving the lives of their patients. Our collective efforts in understanding and addressing neck pain can pave the way for enhanced treatment strategies and, ultimately, a brighter future for those affected by this pervasive condition.

*Sincerely,*

*Branko Weitzmann*

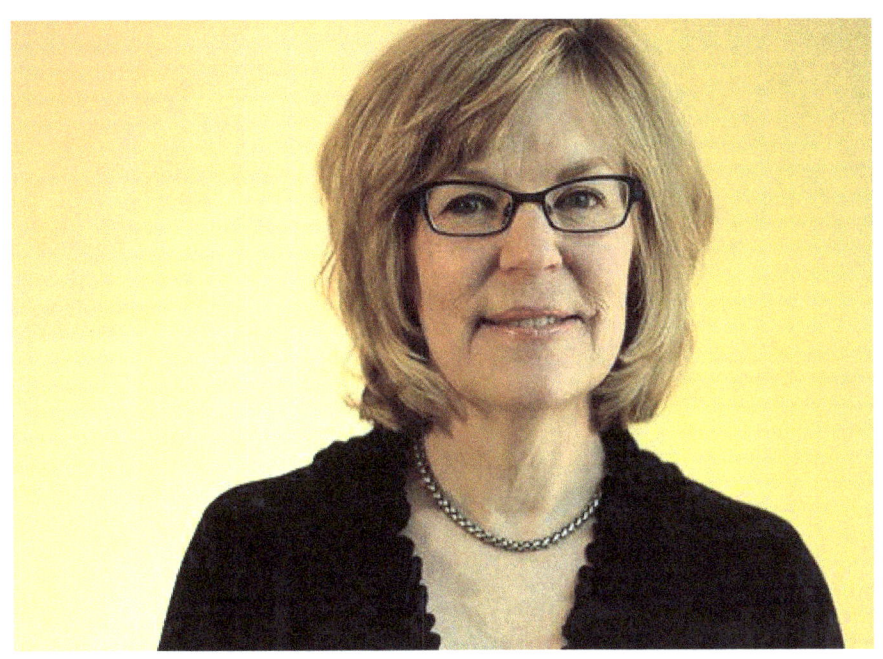

*"Has nobody noticed the embarrassing fact that science is about to clone a human being, but it still can't cure the pain of a bad neck?"*
– Marni Jackson

# Chapter 1

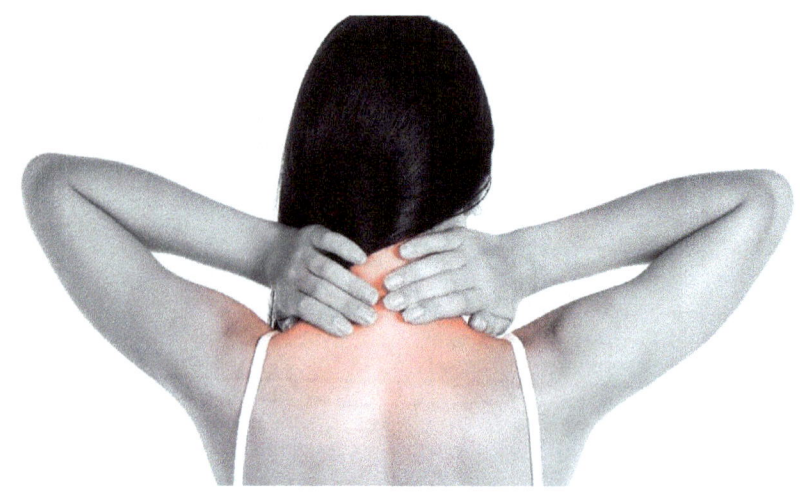

## Understanding Neck Pain

### 1. Anatomy of the neck

The neck, also known as the cervical spine, is a remarkable and complex structure that plays a crucial role in supporting the head, facilitating movement, and protecting the delicate spinal cord. An understanding of the anatomy of the neck is fundamental to comprehending the mechanisms underlying neck pain and the diverse factors that can contribute to this common and often debilitating condition.

The cervical spine consists of seven vertebrae, labeled C1 through C7, which form the bony framework of the neck. These vertebrae are connected by intervertebral discs, fibrous structures that provide cushioning and flexibility, allowing for a wide range of motion in the neck. The cervical spine is further supported and stabilized by ligaments, muscles, and tendons, which work in concert to facilitate movement while maintaining structural integrity.

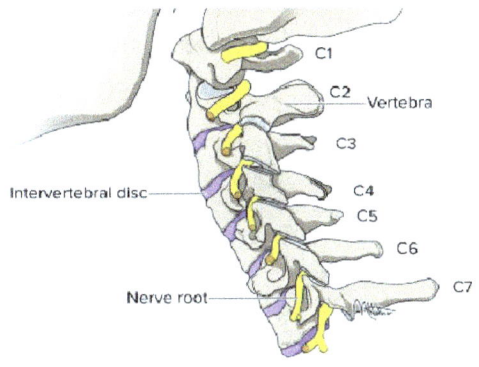

The spinal cord, a vital component of the central nervous system, runs through the vertebral canal formed by the cervical vertebrae. This intricate bundle of nerves serves as the primary conduit for transmitting sensory and motor signals between the brain and the rest of the body. The spinal cord is encased and protected by the vertebrae and is surrounded by protective layers of tissue, including the meninges.

The neck is also home to a network of blood vessels, including the carotid arteries, which supply oxygenated blood to the brain, and the jugular veins, which carry deoxygenated blood away from the brain. These vascular structures are essential for sustaining the metabolic needs of the brain and are intricately intertwined with the anatomical landscape of the neck.

The intricate interplay of bones, discs, ligaments, muscles, tendons, nerves, and blood vessels within the neck creates a dynamic and resilient structure capable of supporting the head and facilitating a wide range of movements, including flexion, extension, rotation, and lateral bending. However, this remarkable flexibility and mobility also render the neck susceptible to a variety of stressors and potential sources of pain.

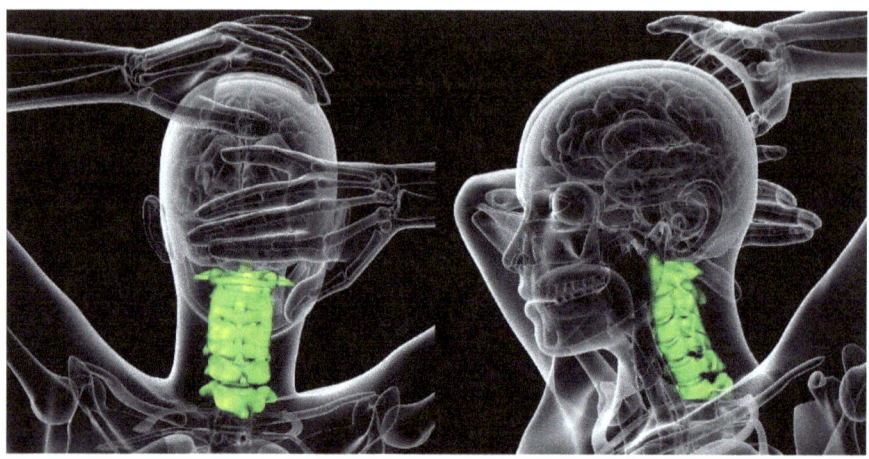

One of the most common sources of neck pain is musculoskeletal in nature, often stemming from strain or tension in the muscles and soft tissues of the neck. Prolonged periods of poor posture, repetitive movements, and excessive strain on the neck muscles can lead to discomfort and stiffness. Additionally, injuries such as whiplash, which can occur during sudden acceleration-deceleration events, may result in damage to the muscles, ligaments, and discs of the neck, leading to acute or chronic pain.

Degenerative changes in the cervical spine, such as osteoarthritis, disc degeneration, and spinal stenosis, can also contribute to neck pain. These age-related changes can lead to the narrowing of the spinal canal, compression of nerve roots, and the formation of bone spurs, all of which can elicit pain and discomfort in the neck and surrounding areas.

Furthermore, the neck can be a site of referred pain originating from other structures, such as the shoulders, upper back, or jaw. Dysfunction in these areas can manifest as pain in the neck, highlighting the interconnected nature of the musculoskeletal system and the potential for pain to radiate across anatomical boundaries.

In some cases, neck pain may be linked to underlying medical conditions, such as cervical radiculopathy, in which a nerve root in the cervical spine is compressed or inflamed, leading to pain, weakness, and sensory changes that radiate into the upper extremities. Additionally, rare but serious conditions, such as tumors or infections affecting the structures of the neck, may present with neck pain as a prominent symptom, underscoring the importance of a thorough evaluation by healthcare professionals when neck pain is persistent or accompanied by concerning symptoms.

Understanding the intricate anatomy of the neck provides a foundation for comprehending the diverse array of factors that can contribute to neck pain. By recognizing the interconnectedness of the bones, muscles, nerves, and blood vessels within the neck, we gain insight into the potential sources of discomfort and the complex interplay of biological, mechanical, and physiological factors that underlie neck pain.

In the pursuit of addressing neck pain, a comprehensive understanding of the anatomy of the neck serves as a cornerstone for developing effective strategies for prevention, management, and treatment. By integrating this knowledge into clinical practice, healthcare professionals can tailor their approach to address the unique needs of individuals grappling with neck pain, fostering a more personalized and targeted approach to care.

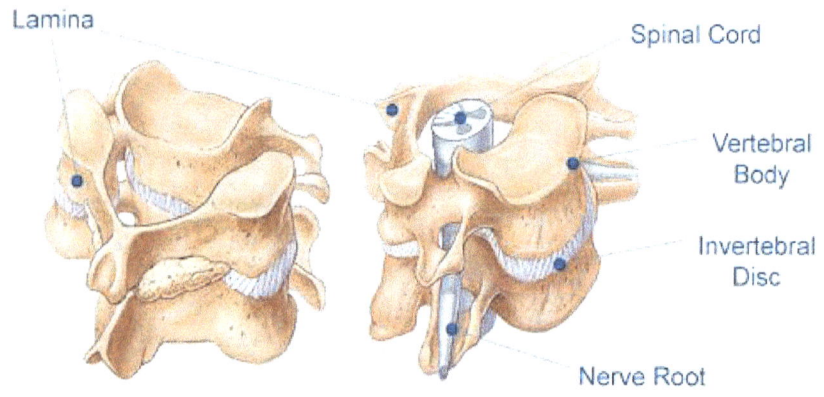

Moreover, individuals affected by neck pain can benefit from gaining insight into the anatomical underpinnings of their condition, empowering them to make informed decisions about their care and take proactive steps to promote neck health and well-being. By fostering a deeper understanding of the anatomy of the neck, we can enhance the dialogue between patients and healthcare professionals, promoting collaboration and shared decision-making in the pursuit of optimal neck pain management.

In conclusion, the anatomy of the neck is a marvel of biological engineering, encompassing a complex interplay of bones, muscles, nerves, and blood vessels that support mobility, protect vital structures, and facilitate sensory and motor function. By delving into the intricacies of the cervical spine, we gain a deeper appreciation for the factors that can contribute to neck pain and the diverse mechanisms underlying this common and multifaceted condition. This understanding serves as a foundation for advancing our approach to addressing neck pain, fostering a more holistic, personalized, and effective approach to care for individuals affected by this pervasive condition.

## 2. Common causes of neck pain

Neck pain is a prevalent and multifaceted condition that can stem from a variety of sources, ranging from everyday activities to underlying medical conditions. Understanding the common causes of neck pain is essential for recognizing the diverse factors that can contribute to this often debilitating issue and for developing targeted strategies for prevention and management.

Muscle Strain and Tension: One of the most frequent causes of neck pain is muscle strain and tension. Prolonged periods of poor posture, such as hunching over a computer or slouching while using a smartphone, can place excessive stress on the muscles of the neck and upper back, leading to discomfort and stiffness. Additionally, activities that involve repetitive movements or heavy lifting can strain the neck muscles, contributing to pain and reduced mobility.

## Muscle Strain

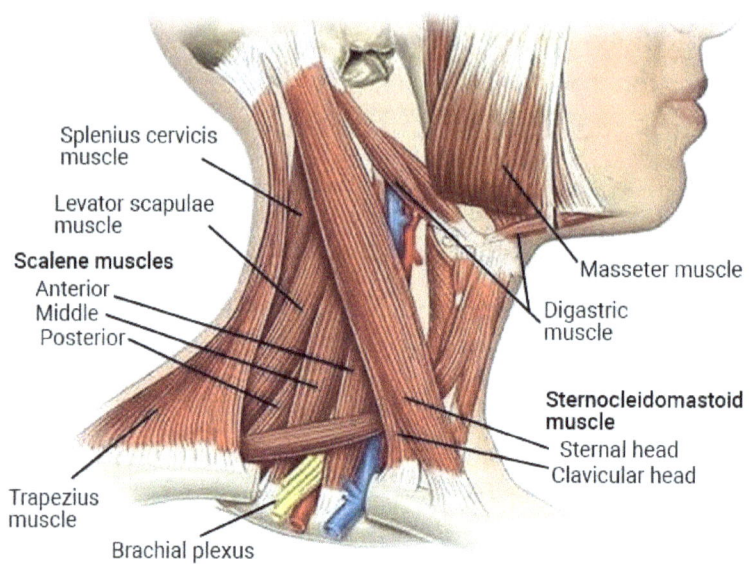

Splenius cervicis muscle
Levator scapulae muscle
**Scalene muscles**
Anterior
Middle
Posterior
Trapezius muscle
Brachial plexus
Masseter muscle
Digastric muscle
**Sternocleidomastoid muscle**
Sternal head
Clavicular head

<u>Whiplash Injuries:</u> Whiplash is a common injury that occurs when the head is suddenly jerked forward and then backward, often as a result of motor vehicle accidents, sports-related collisions, or physical assaults. This rapid and forceful movement can cause damage to the muscles, ligaments, and discs of the neck, leading to acute or chronic neck pain, as well as other symptoms such as headaches, dizziness, and cognitive difficulties.

<u>Degenerative Changes:</u> Age-related degenerative changes in the cervical spine, such as osteoarthritis, disc degeneration, and spinal stenosis, can contribute

to neck pain. These changes can lead to the narrowing of the spinal canal, compression of nerve roots, and the formation of bone spurs, all of which can elicit pain and discomfort in the neck and surrounding areas. Over time, the wear and tear on the structures of the neck can result in chronic pain and reduced mobility.

Poor Ergonomics: The way we position our bodies during various activities, including working at a desk, using electronic devices, and engaging in physical tasks, can significantly impact the health of our necks. Poor ergonomics, such as an improperly adjusted workstation, inadequate support for the head and neck, and repetitive movements in awkward positions, can contribute to muscle strain, tension, and discomfort in the neck.

Referred Pain: Dysfunction in other areas of the body, such as the shoulders, upper back, or jaw, can manifest as pain in the neck. Referred pain occurs when pain originating from one area is perceived in another location, highlighting the interconnected nature of the musculoskeletal system. For example, a shoulder injury or tension in the upper back muscles can lead to pain that radiates into the neck, complicating the diagnosis and management of neck pain.

Cervical Radiculopathy: Cervical radiculopathy occurs when a nerve root in the cervical spine is compressed or inflamed, leading to pain, weakness, and sensory changes that radiate into the upper extremities. This condition can result from herniated discs, bone spurs, or other degenerative changes in the cervical spine, and it can cause significant discomfort and functional impairment.

Underlying Medical Conditions: In some cases, neck pain may be linked to underlying medical conditions, such as infections, tumors, or inflammatory disorders affecting the structures of the neck. While these conditions are relatively rare, they can present with neck pain as a prominent symptom, underscoring the importance of a thorough evaluation by healthcare professionals when neck pain is persistent or accompanied by concerning symptoms.

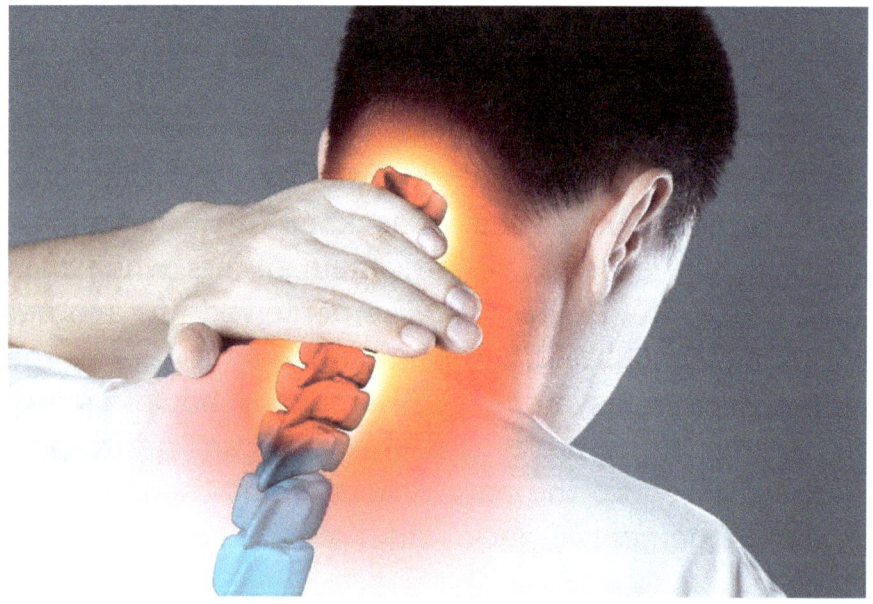

Psychological and Emotional Factors: Psychological and emotional factors, such as stress, anxiety, and depression, can influence the experience of neck pain. Chronic stress and emotional distress can contribute to muscle tension and exacerbate existing neck pain, creating a complex interplay between physical and psychological well-being.

Understanding the common causes of neck pain provides a foundation for recognizing the diverse factors that can contribute to this pervasive condition. By acknowledging the multifaceted nature of neck pain, healthcare professionals and individuals affected by this issue can develop a more comprehensive and targeted approach to prevention, management, and treatment.

In the pursuit of addressing neck pain, a holistic understanding of the common causes of neck pain serves as a cornerstone for fostering effective strategies for prevention and management. By integrating this knowledge into clinical practice, healthcare professionals can tailor their approach to address the unique needs of individuals grappling with neck pain, fostering a more personalized and targeted approach to care.

Moreover, individuals affected by neck pain can benefit from gaining insight into the common causes of their condition, empowering them to make informed decisions about their care and take proactive steps to promote neck health and well-being. By fostering a deeper understanding of the common causes of neck pain, we can enhance the dialogue between patients and healthcare professionals, promoting collaboration and shared decision-making in the pursuit of optimal neck pain management.

In conclusion, the common causes of neck pain encompass a diverse array of factors, including muscle strain, whiplash injuries, degenerative changes, poor ergonomics, referred pain, cervical radiculopathy, underlying medical conditions, and psychological and emotional factors. By delving into the multifaceted nature of neck pain, we gain a deeper appreciation for the factors that can contribute to discomfort and the complex interplay of biological, mechanical, and psychological factors that underlie this prevalent condition. This understanding serves as a foundation for advancing our approach to addressing neck pain, fostering a more holistic, personalized, and effective approach to care for individuals affected by this pervasive issue.

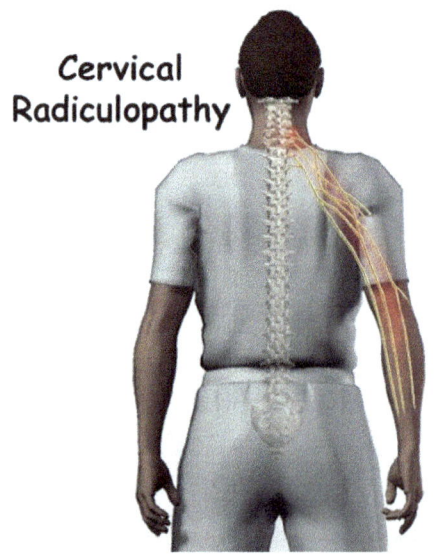

**Cervical Radiculopathy**

### 3. Types of neck pain (acute, chronic, etc.)
Neck pain is a common ailment that can be caused by a variety of factors, including poor posture, muscle

strain, injury, or underlying health conditions. Understanding the different types of neck pain can help individuals and healthcare professionals identify the underlying causes and determine the most effective treatment approaches. In this article, we will explore several types of neck pain, including acute neck pain, chronic neck pain, and other specific conditions that can affect the neck.

## Acute Neck Pain:

Acute neck pain is characterized by sudden onset and typically lasts for a relatively short period of time, usually a few days to a few weeks. This type of neck pain is often caused by muscle strain or injury, such as whiplash from a car accident or a sudden jerking motion during physical activity. Acute neck pain can also be the result of poor posture, such as hunching over a computer for an extended period of time. Individuals with acute neck pain may experience symptoms such as stiffness, sharp pain, and limited range of motion. Treatment for acute neck pain often involves rest, gentle stretching exercises, over-the-counter pain medication, and applying ice or heat to the affected area.

## Chronic Neck Pain:

Chronic neck pain is characterized by persistent or recurring pain in the neck that lasts for 12 weeks or longer. This type of neck pain can be caused by a variety of factors, including underlying health conditions, such as arthritis, degenerative disc disease, or cervical spondylosis. Chronic neck pain can also be the result of long-term poor posture, repetitive strain, or unresolved acute neck pain. Individuals with chronic neck pain may experience symptoms such as dull aching, stiffness, and discomfort that may radiate to the shoulders, arms, or head. Treatment for chronic neck pain often involves a combination of physical therapy, pain management techniques, and in some cases, surgical intervention.

## Cervical Radiculopathy:

Cervical radiculopathy, also known as a pinched nerve, occurs when a nerve in the neck is compressed or irritated, leading to pain, weakness, or numbness that radiates down the arm. This condition can be caused by a herniated disc, bone spurs, or spinal stenosis in the cervical spine. Individuals with cervical radiculopathy may experience symptoms such as shooting pain, tingling, or weakness in the arm or hand on one side of the body. Treatment for cervical radiculopathy may include physical therapy, medication, epidural steroid injections, or in severe cases, surgical decompression of the affected nerve.

## Cervical Spondylosis:

Cervical spondylosis, also known as neck arthritis, is a degenerative condition that affects the cervical spine as a result of age-related changes, such as the formation of bone spurs and the breakdown of spinal discs. Individuals with cervical spondylosis may experience symptoms such as neck pain, stiffness, and reduced range of motion. In some cases, cervical spondylosis can lead to the compression of spinal nerves, resulting in symptoms such as radiating pain, weakness, or numbness in the arms. Treatment for cervical spondylosis may include physical therapy, medication, and in severe cases, surgical intervention to relieve pressure on the affected nerves.

## Whiplash:

Whiplash is a neck injury that occurs when the head is suddenly jerked backward and then forward, such as during a car accident. This rapid motion can cause damage to the soft tissues in the neck, leading to symptoms such as neck pain, stiffness, headaches, and in some cases, cognitive or psychological symptoms. Treatment for whiplash may include rest, physical therapy, pain medication, and in some cases, interventions to address associated symptoms, such as cognitive behavioral therapy for anxiety or depression.

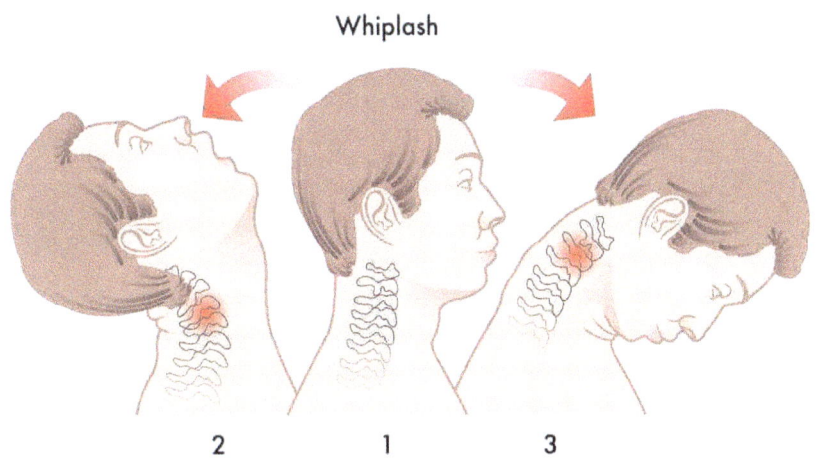

Whiplash

In conclusion, neck pain can manifest in various forms, ranging from acute muscle strain to chronic degenerative conditions. Understanding the different types of neck pain and their underlying causes is essential for accurate diagnosis and effective treatment. Individuals experiencing neck pain should seek medical evaluation to determine the most appropriate course of action for their specific condition.

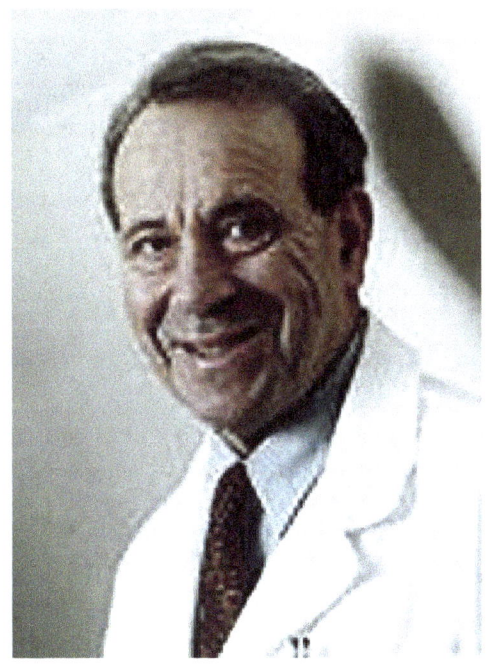

*"I've been studying neck pain for the last 50 years of my life and if anyone says they know where low back pain comes from, they're full of s\*\*t."*

– Alf Nachemson

# Chapter 2

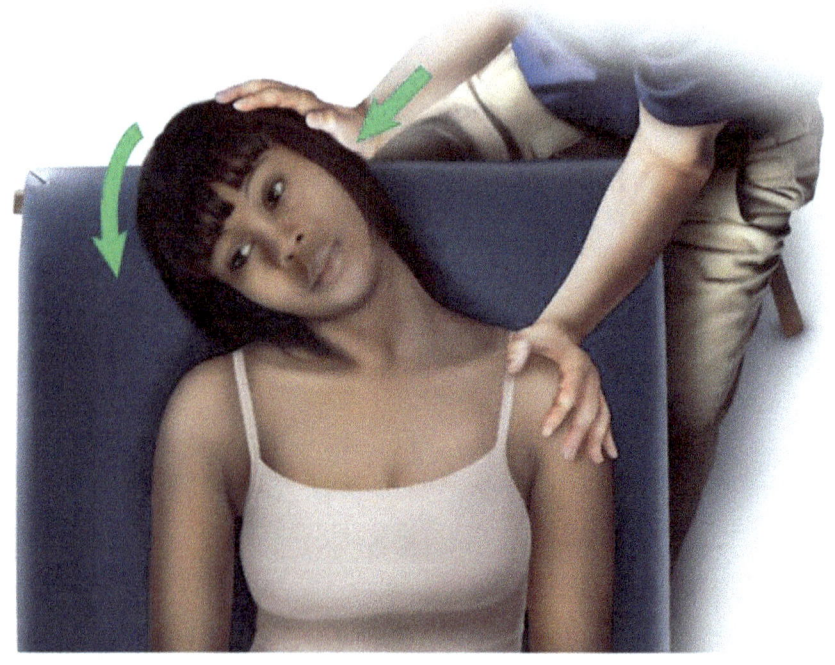

## Diagnosis and Assessment

### 1. Medical history and physical examination

When a patient presents with neck pain, a comprehensive medical history and physical examination are essential for accurately diagnosing the underlying cause and determining the most appropriate treatment plan. In this article, we will explore the importance of medical history and physical examination in the assessment of neck pain, including key components and considerations for healthcare professionals.

## Medical History:

Obtaining a thorough medical history is the first step in evaluating a patient with neck pain. The medical history should include detailed information about the onset and duration of the neck pain, any precipitating factors or traumatic events, and a description of the nature and location of the pain. Additionally, healthcare professionals should inquire about any previous treatments or interventions for neck pain, as well as the patient's medical and surgical history, including any underlying health conditions or medications that may be relevant to the current complaint.

Furthermore, it is important to assess the impact of neck pain on the patient's daily activities, work, and quality of life. Inquiring about any associated symptoms, such as radiating pain, numbness, weakness, or changes in bowel or bladder function, can provide valuable insights into the potential underlying causes of the neck pain. Additionally, healthcare professionals should ask about any red flag symptoms, such as fever, unexplained weight loss, or a history of cancer, as these may indicate more serious underlying conditions that require further evaluation.

## Physical Examination:

A comprehensive physical examination is crucial for evaluating neck pain and identifying any physical findings that may help elucidate the underlying cause. The physical examination should include an assessment of the patient's posture, range of motion, and palpation of the neck and surrounding structures. Healthcare professionals should also evaluate for any signs of inflammation, such as redness, swelling, or warmth, which may indicate an acute inflammatory process.

Assessment of neurological function is an important component of the physical examination, as it can help identify any nerve-related symptoms or deficits. This may include testing for strength, sensation, reflexes, and specific maneuvers to assess nerve root compression or irritation. Additionally, special tests, such as Spurling's test or the shoulder abduction test, may be performed to further evaluate for cervical radiculopathy or other specific conditions.

Furthermore, the physical examination should include an assessment of the cervical spine for any structural abnormalities, such as misalignment, tenderness, or abnormal curvatures. Healthcare professionals should also evaluate for any signs of muscle spasm, trigger points, or myofascial pain, which may be indicative of muscular or soft tissue involvement in the neck pain.

## Diagnostic Considerations:

In addition to the medical history and physical examination, healthcare professionals may consider further diagnostic studies to aid in the evaluation of neck pain. This may include imaging studies, such as X-rays, magnetic resonance imaging (MRI), or computed tomography (CT) scans, to assess the bony and soft tissue structures of the cervical spine. These studies can help identify structural abnormalities, such as fractures, degenerative changes, or herniated discs, that may be contributing to the neck pain.

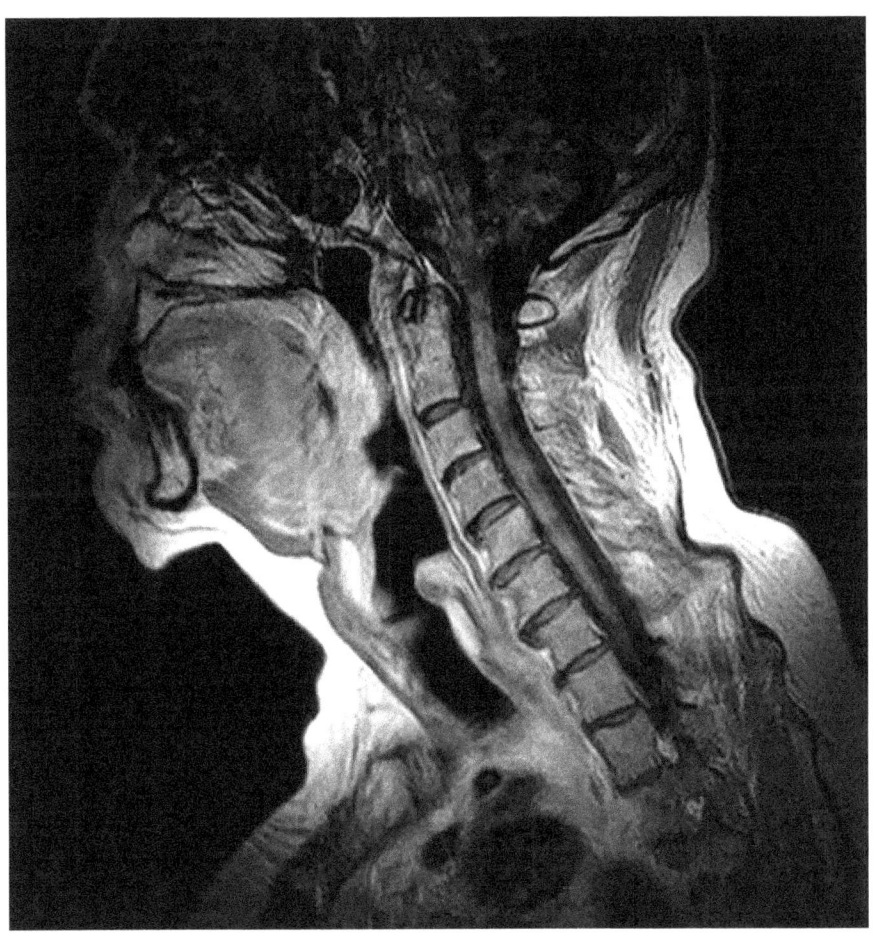

Furthermore, diagnostic studies, such as electromyography (EMG) or nerve conduction studies, may be considered to assess for nerve-related symptoms or deficits. These studies can help localize the site of nerve compression or irritation and provide valuable information for treatment planning.

In some cases, additional laboratory tests, such as complete blood count (CBC), erythrocyte sedimentation rate (ESR), or C-reactive protein (CRP) may be ordered to assess for signs of inflammation or underlying systemic conditions that may be contributing to the neck pain.

## Treatment Planning:

Based on the findings from the medical history, physical examination, and any additional diagnostic studies, healthcare professionals can develop a comprehensive treatment plan for neck pain. This may include a combination of conservative measures, such as physical therapy, medication, and lifestyle modifications, as well as interventions, such as injections or surgical procedures, for more severe or refractory cases.

Furthermore, patient education and self-management strategies are important components of the treatment plan, as they can empower patients to take an active role in managing their neck pain and preventing future recurrences. Healthcare professionals should provide guidance on ergonomic principles, posture correction, and exercises to improve strength, flexibility, and overall neck health.

In conclusion, a thorough medical history and physical examination are essential for evaluating neck pain and determining the most appropriate course of action for each individual patient. By carefully assessing the patient's symptoms, physical findings, and any relevant diagnostic studies, healthcare professionals can develop a tailored treatment plan that addresses the underlying cause of the neck pain and helps patients achieve optimal outcomes.

## 2. Imaging and diagnostic tests

Imaging and diagnostic tests play a crucial role in the evaluation of neck pain, aiding healthcare professionals in identifying the underlying causes, assessing the severity of the condition, and determining the most appropriate treatment plan. In this article, we will explore the various imaging modalities and diagnostic tests commonly used in the assessment of neck pain, including their indications, benefits, and considerations for healthcare professionals.

### X-rays:

X-rays are often the initial imaging modality used to evaluate neck pain, as they provide detailed images of the bony structures of the cervical spine. X-rays can help identify fractures, dislocations, degenerative changes, and other bony abnormalities that may be contributing to the neck pain. Additionally, X-rays can assess the alignment of the cervical spine, the integrity of the vertebral bodies, and the presence of bone spurs or osteophytes.

X-rays are particularly useful in the evaluation of traumatic injuries, such as whiplash-associated disorders or fractures resulting from falls or accidents. They are also valuable in assessing degenerative conditions, such as cervical spondylosis or osteoarthritis, which may be contributing to the patient's neck pain. Furthermore, X-rays can be used to monitor the progression of certain conditions over time, such as the development of spinal instability or the healing of fractures.

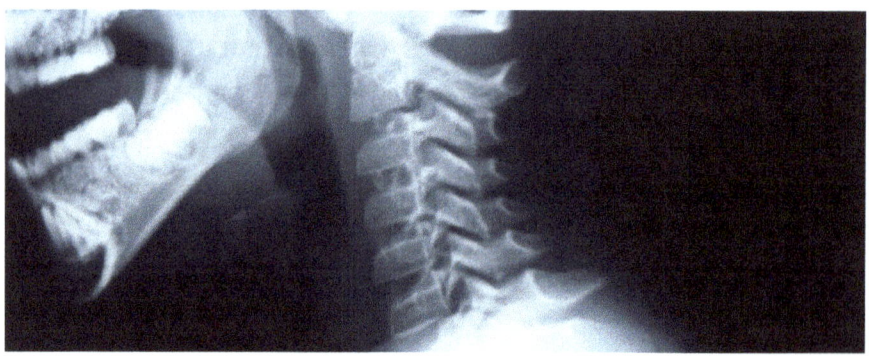

## Computed Tomography (CT) Scan:

CT scans provide detailed cross-sectional images of the cervical spine, offering a more comprehensive assessment of the bony structures, soft tissues, and neural elements. CT scans are particularly useful in the evaluation of complex fractures, spinal stenosis, and other conditions that may not be adequately visualized on X-rays alone. Additionally, CT scans can help identify the precise location and extent of bony abnormalities, such as fractures, dislocations, or bone spurs, that may be contributing to the patient's neck pain.

CT scans are also valuable in the preoperative planning of surgical interventions, as they can provide detailed anatomical information and aid in the identification of potential surgical targets. Furthermore, CT myelography, which involves the injection of contrast dye into the spinal canal prior to CT scanning, can be used to assess for nerve root compression, spinal cord abnormalities, or other soft tissue lesions that may be contributing to the patient's symptoms.

## Magnetic Resonance Imaging (MRI):

MRI is a powerful imaging modality that provides detailed images of the soft tissues, including the spinal cord, nerve roots, intervertebral discs, and surrounding musculature. MRI is particularly valuable in the evaluation of conditions such as herniated discs, spinal cord compression, spinal tumors, and inflammatory or infectious processes that may be contributing to the patient's neck pain. Additionally, MRI can help identify soft tissue injuries, such as ligamentous or muscular strains, that may not be visualized on X-rays or CT scans.

Furthermore, MRI can provide valuable information about the vascularity and perfusion of soft tissues, aiding in the assessment of conditions such as cervical radiculopathy, myelopathy, or inflammatory disorders. Functional MRI techniques, such as diffusion-weighted imaging or dynamic contrast-enhanced MRI, can also be used to assess for changes in tissue microstructure, blood flow, or metabolic activity that may be indicative of specific pathological processes.

## Electrodiagnostic Studies:

Electrodiagnostic studies, such as electromyography (EMG) and nerve conduction studies (NCS), can be valuable in the assessment of nerve-related symptoms or deficits in patients with neck pain. EMG involves the insertion of fine needle electrodes into specific muscles to assess for signs of denervation, muscle activation patterns, and the presence of abnormal spontaneous activity. NCS involves the application of surface electrodes and mild electrical stimulation to assess the conduction of nerve impulses along specific nerve pathways.

These studies can help localize the site of nerve compression or irritation, assess the severity of nerve dysfunction, and differentiate between radicular symptoms and other musculoskeletal or systemic conditions. Additionally, electrodiagnostic studies can provide valuable information for treatment planning, prognostication, and monitoring the progression of nerve-related conditions over time.

## Other Diagnostic Tests:

In addition to imaging studies and electrodiagnostic tests, other diagnostic studies may be considered in the evaluation of neck pain, depending on the specific clinical presentation and suspected underlying causes. These may include laboratory tests, such as complete blood count (CBC), erythrocyte sedimentation rate (ESR), C-reactive protein (CRP), and specific serological tests for autoimmune or infectious conditions that may be contributing to the neck pain.

Furthermore, diagnostic injections, such as facet joint injections, medial branch blocks, or selective nerve root blocks, may be used to assess the source of the patient's pain and determine the potential efficacy of targeted interventions, such as radiofrequency ablation or spinal fusion surgery. These diagnostic injections can help differentiate between pain originating from specific structures in the cervical spine and guide the selection of appropriate treatment modalities.

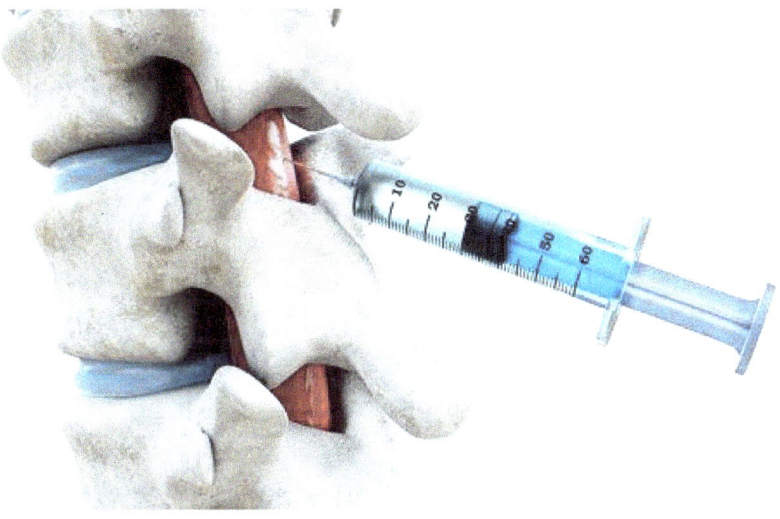

In conclusion, imaging and diagnostic tests play a critical role in the evaluation of neck pain, providing valuable information about the underlying causes, severity, and potential treatment options. By carefully selecting and interpreting the appropriate imaging modalities and diagnostic tests, healthcare professionals can develop a comprehensive understanding of the patient's condition and develop a tailored treatment plan that addresses the specific needs and goals of each individual patient.

## 3. Assessing the impact on daily life and function

Neck pain can have a significant impact on an individual's daily life and function, affecting their ability to perform routine activities, work, and engage in recreational pursuits. Understanding the impact of neck pain on various aspects of daily living is essential for healthcare professionals to develop comprehensive treatment plans that address the specific needs and goals of each patient. In this article, we will explore the assessment of the impact of neck pain on daily life and function, including key considerations and strategies for healthcare professionals.

## Physical Function:

Assessing the impact of neck pain on physical function involves evaluating the patient's ability to perform activities of daily living, such as dressing, grooming, and household chores, as well as more physically demanding tasks, such as lifting, carrying, or participating in sports or recreational activities. Healthcare professionals should inquire about any limitations in range of motion, strength, or endurance that may be affecting the patient's ability to engage in these activities.

Furthermore, it is important to assess the impact of neck pain on posture, balance, and coordination, as these factors can influence the risk of falls, musculoskeletal strain, and overall physical well-being. Healthcare professionals may use standardized assessment tools, such as the Neck Disability Index (NDI) or the Patient-Specific Functional Scale (PSFS), to quantify the impact of neck pain on physical function and monitor changes over time.

## Work and Productivity:

Neck pain can significantly impact an individual's ability to work and be productive, leading to absenteeism, presenteeism, and reduced job performance. Healthcare professionals should assess the patient's occupational demands, including the physical requirements of their job, the ergonomic factors in their work environment, and any specific challenges related to their neck pain.

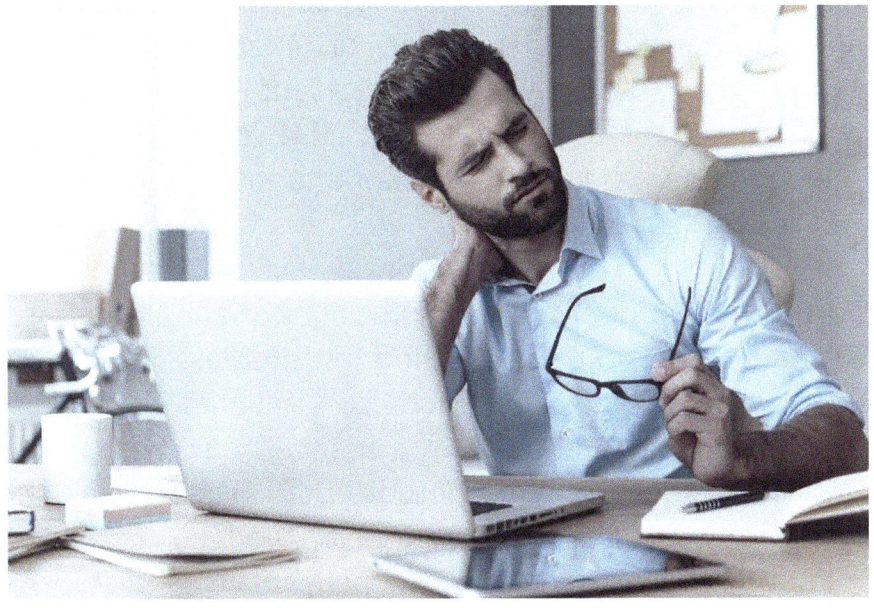

Furthermore, it is important to inquire about the impact of neck pain on work-related tasks, such as typing, lifting, or prolonged sitting or standing, as well as any accommodations or modifications that may be necessary to support the patient's return to work or continued employment. Healthcare professionals may collaborate with occupational health specialists, physical therapists, or vocational rehabilitation experts to develop tailored strategies for managing neck pain in the workplace and promoting a safe and productive work environment.

## Psychosocial Well-being:

Neck pain can have a profound impact on an individual's psychosocial well-being, leading to emotional distress, social isolation, and reduced quality of life. Healthcare professionals should assess the patient's emotional responses to neck pain, including feelings of frustration, anxiety, depression, or fear of exacerbating their symptoms. Additionally, it is important to inquire about the impact of neck pain on the patient's social relationships, leisure activities, and overall sense of well-being.

Furthermore, healthcare professionals should assess for any maladaptive coping strategies, such as avoidance of physical activity, reliance on pain medication, or excessive reliance on healthcare providers, which may perpetuate the cycle of disability and distress. Collaborative care models, involving mental health professionals, pain psychologists, or support groups, can be valuable in addressing the psychosocial impact of neck pain and promoting resilience, self-efficacy, and adaptive coping strategies.

## Sleep and Rest:

Neck pain can significantly impact an individual's sleep quality and overall restfulness, leading to fatigue, irritability, and impaired cognitive function. Healthcare professionals should assess the patient's sleep patterns, including the duration, quality, and efficiency of their sleep, as well as any specific factors that may be contributing to sleep disturbances, such as pain, discomfort, or anxiety.

Furthermore, it is important to inquire about the patient's use of sleep aids, such as medications, pillows, or positional strategies, and assess the impact of these interventions on their overall sleep hygiene. Healthcare professionals may provide guidance on sleep hygiene principles, relaxation techniques, and pain management strategies to promote restful sleep and improve the patient's overall energy levels and daytime functioning.

## Functional Goals and Expectations:
Assessing the impact of neck pain on daily life and function should also involve a discussion of the patient's functional goals and expectations for treatment. Healthcare professionals should inquire about the specific activities, roles, and responsibilities that are most meaningful to the patient and identify any barriers or challenges that may be hindering their ability to achieve these goals.

Furthermore, it is important to collaborate with the patient to develop realistic and achievable functional goals, such as returning to work, participating in recreational activities, or improving overall physical fitness, and develop a tailored treatment plan that addresses these specific goals. Shared decision-making models, involving the patient as an active participant in their care, can help promote engagement, motivation, and adherence to treatment recommendations.

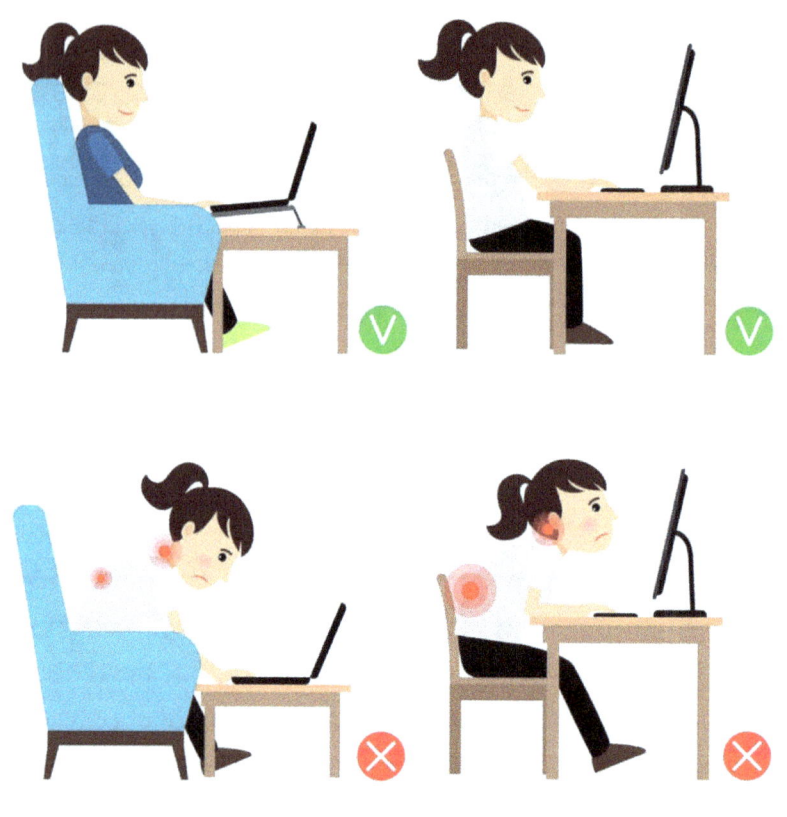

In conclusion, assessing the impact of neck pain on daily life and function is essential for healthcare professionals to develop comprehensive treatment plans that address the specific needs and goals of each patient. By carefully evaluating the physical, occupational, psychosocial, and functional aspects of neck pain, healthcare professionals can develop tailored strategies for managing neck pain and promoting optimal outcomes for their patients. Collaborative care models, involving multidisciplinary teams and patient-centered approaches, can help address the complex and multifaceted impact of neck pain on daily living and function.

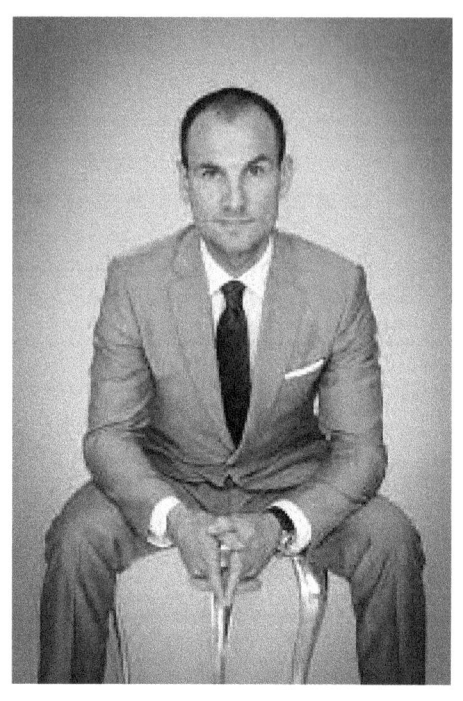

*"For decades we have scanned, screened and tested. Spines have been cut, carved and fixated. However, on our seemingly never-ending quest to find the pathoanatomical 'Holy Grail' of pain, we seem to be forgetting something: Our patients are not cars. And we are not mechanics."*
– Jørgen Jevne

# Chapter 3

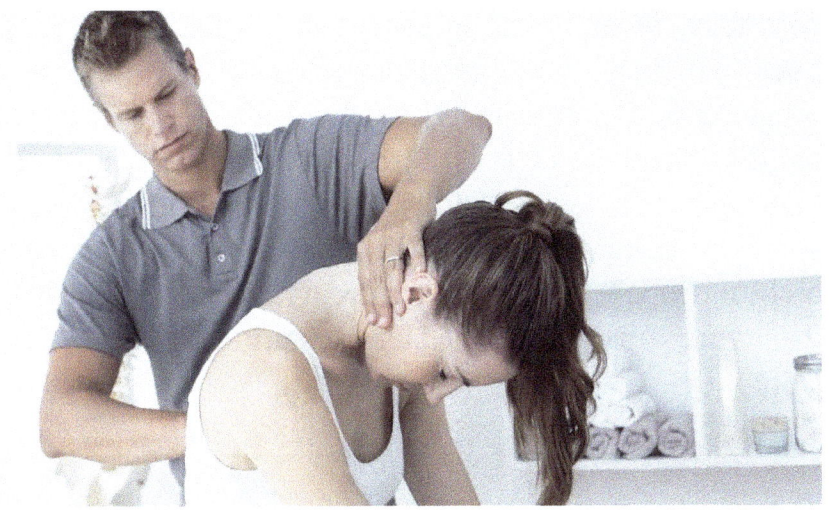

## Non-Specific Neck Pain

### 1. Exploring non-specific neck pain

Non-specific neck pain is a common musculoskeletal condition characterized by discomfort, stiffness, or tension in the cervical region without a specific identifiable cause. This type of neck pain accounts for a significant proportion of neck pain presentations in clinical practice and can have a substantial impact on an individual's quality of life and functional abilities. In this article, we will explore non-specific neck pain, including its clinical presentation, potential contributing factors, diagnostic considerations, and management strategies.

### Clinical Presentation:

Non-specific neck pain is typically described as a diffuse discomfort or stiffness in the cervical region, often without a clear precipitating event or identifiable pathology. Patients may report sensations of tension, soreness, or achiness in the neck, shoulders, or upper back, which may be exacerbated by certain movements or sustained postures. The pain may be unilateral or bilateral and can radiate to the shoulders, arms, or head in some cases. Additionally, individuals with non-specific neck pain may experience limitations in range of motion, particularly with activities such as turning the head, looking up or down, or tilting the head to the side.

## Contributing Factors:

Several factors may contribute to the development of non-specific neck pain, including poor posture, prolonged sitting or standing, repetitive movements, muscle imbalances, and psychosocial stressors. Occupational factors, such as prolonged computer use, heavy lifting, or repetitive overhead work, can also contribute to the onset or exacerbation of non-specific neck pain. Additionally, psychosocial factors, such as anxiety, depression, or maladaptive coping strategies, may influence the perception and experience of neck pain, leading to increased disability and reduced quality of life.

## Diagnostic Considerations:

Diagnosing non-specific neck pain involves a comprehensive assessment of the patient's medical history, physical examination findings, and exclusion of specific underlying pathologies. Healthcare professionals should inquire about the onset and duration of the neck pain, any precipitating events, and the impact of the pain on the patient's daily activities and function. Additionally, it is important to assess for any red flag symptoms, such as fever, unexplained weight loss, or a history of cancer, which may warrant further investigation for specific underlying causes.

Physical examination findings in non-specific neck pain may include localized tenderness, muscle spasm, reduced range of motion, and the absence of neurological deficits or signs of serious pathology. Diagnostic imaging, such as X-rays, CT scans, or MRI, may be considered if there are atypical features, progressive neurological symptoms, or a lack of improvement with conservative management. However, it is important to note that imaging findings in non-specific neck pain may not always correlate with the severity of symptoms or functional limitations.

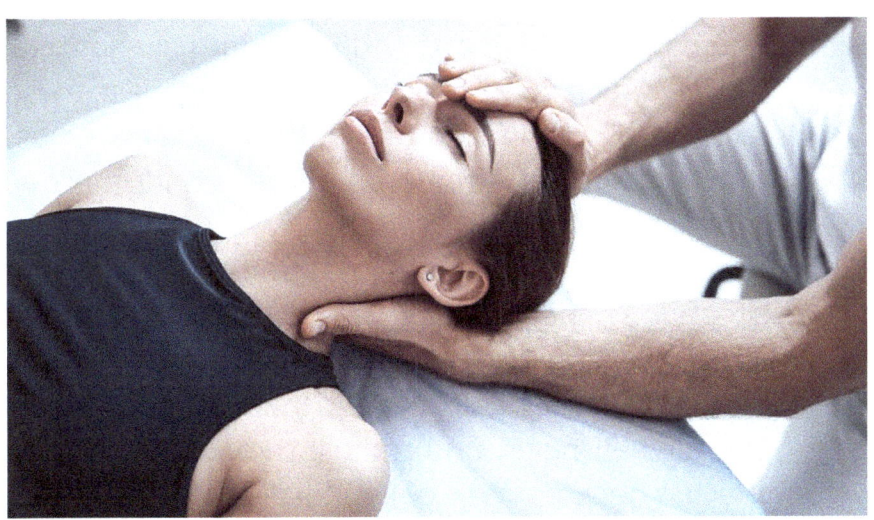

## Management Strategies:

The management of non-specific neck pain often involves a multimodal approach aimed at addressing pain, improving function, and addressing contributing factors. Conservative treatment options may include:

1. Physical Therapy: Targeted exercises, manual therapy, and postural education can help improve strength, flexibility, and overall neck health. Additionally, ergonomic assessments and modifications may be recommended to optimize the patient's work or home environment.

2. Pain Management: Over-the-counter or prescription medications, such as nonsteroidal anti-inflammatory drugs (NSAIDs), muscle relaxants, or analgesics, may be used to alleviate pain and improve the patient's comfort.

3. Psychosocial Support: Addressing psychosocial factors, such as stress management, relaxation techniques, and cognitive-behavioral strategies, can help reduce emotional distress and improve coping skills.

4. Lifestyle Modifications: Encouraging regular physical activity, proper ergonomics, stress reduction, and healthy sleep habits can support overall well-being and reduce the impact of non-specific neck pain on daily life.

In some cases, complementary therapies, such as acupuncture, massage, or chiropractic care, may be considered as adjunctive treatments for non-specific neck pain. Additionally, healthcare professionals should collaborate with the patient to develop realistic functional goals and monitor progress over time to guide treatment adjustments and optimize outcomes.

In conclusion, non-specific neck pain is a prevalent musculoskeletal condition that can significantly impact an individual's quality of life and functional abilities. Understanding the clinical presentation, contributing factors, diagnostic considerations, and management strategies for non-specific neck pain is essential for healthcare professionals to provide comprehensive care and support for individuals experiencing this common condition. By addressing physical, psychosocial, and lifestyle factors, healthcare professionals can help individuals manage non-specific neck pain and improve their overall well-being and function.

## 2. Contributing factors and risk factors

Non-specific neck pain is a prevalent musculoskeletal condition that can be influenced by a variety of contributing factors and risk factors. Understanding these factors is essential for healthcare professionals to develop comprehensive treatment plans and preventive strategies for individuals experiencing non-specific neck pain. In this article, we will explore the contributing factors and risk factors associated with non-specific neck pain, including their impact on the development, progression, and management of this common condition.

Contributing Factors:

1. <u>Poor Posture</u>: Prolonged periods of sitting or standing with poor posture can place excessive strain on the muscles, ligaments, and joints of the cervical spine, leading to muscle imbalances, tension, and discomfort in the neck and shoulders. Additionally, repetitive activities that involve sustained or awkward postures, such as working at a computer or performing overhead tasks, can contribute to the development of non-specific neck pain.

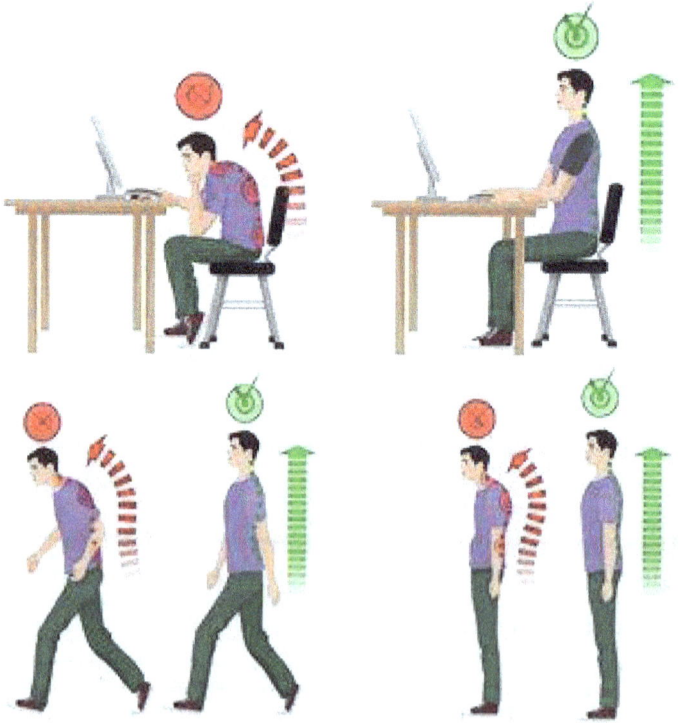

2. Muscular Imbalances: Weakness or tightness in the muscles of the neck, shoulders, and upper back can disrupt the dynamic stability of the cervical spine and alter movement patterns, leading to increased stress on the surrounding tissues and potential discomfort.

3. Repetitive Movements: Engaging in repetitive movements or activities, such as lifting, carrying, or performing manual labor, can strain the muscles and soft tissues of the neck, contributing to the onset or exacerbation of non-specific neck pain.

4. Psychosocial Stressors: Emotional distress, anxiety, depression, and maladaptive coping strategies can influence the perception and experience of neck pain, leading to increased disability, reduced quality of life, and prolonged recovery.

5. Occupational Factors: Work-related factors, such as prolonged computer use, poor ergonomic setups, heavy lifting, repetitive overhead work, and high job demands, can contribute to the development of non-specific neck pain. Additionally, workplace stress, job dissatisfaction, and inadequate rest breaks may further exacerbate the impact of occupational factors on neck pain.

## Risk Factors:

1. Age: The prevalence of non-specific neck pain tends to increase with age, as degenerative changes, wear and tear, and age-related musculoskeletal conditions can contribute to the development of neck discomfort and stiffness.

2. Gender: Studies have suggested that females may be at a higher risk of experiencing non-specific neck pain compared to males, although the reasons for this gender difference are not fully understood and may involve a complex interplay of biological, psychological, and social factors.

3. Physical Fitness: Poor physical fitness, including reduced muscular strength, flexibility, and endurance, may increase the risk of developing non-specific neck pain, as inadequate physical conditioning can compromise the resilience and adaptability of the musculoskeletal system.

4. Smoking: Tobacco use has been associated with an increased risk of musculoskeletal pain, including neck pain. The exact mechanisms underlying this association are not fully elucidated, but it is thought that smoking may affect tissue perfusion, healing processes, and pain modulation systems.

5. Psychosocial Factors: Individuals with high levels of stress, anxiety, depression, or poor coping

skills may be at an increased risk of developing or exacerbating non-specific neck pain. Psychosocial factors can influence pain perception, emotional well-being, and the ability to engage in self-care and healthy lifestyle behaviors.

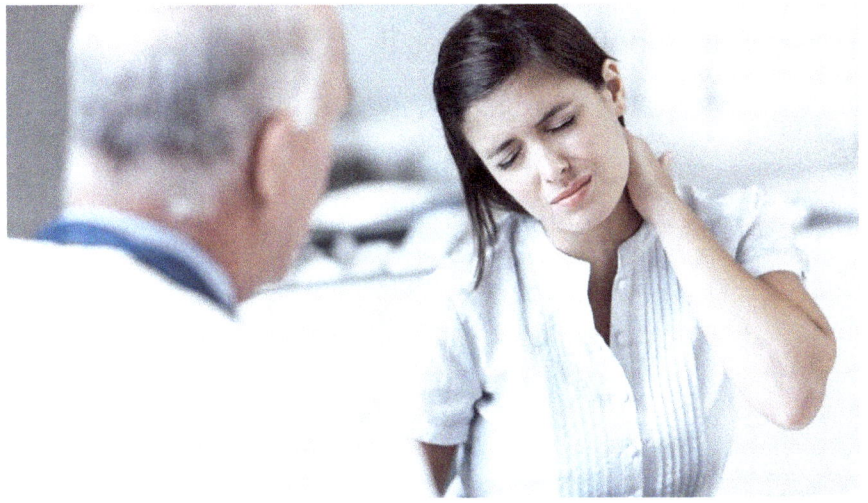

6. <u>Work Environment:</u> Occupational factors, such as prolonged sitting, repetitive tasks, awkward postures, and high job demands, can increase the risk of developing non-specific neck pain. Additionally, job dissatisfaction, poor workplace ergonomics, and inadequate support systems may further contribute to the impact of the work environment on neck pain.

## Management and Prevention:

Addressing contributing factors and risk factors is essential for the management and prevention of non-specific neck pain. Healthcare professionals can implement the following strategies to address these factors:

1. Postural Education: Providing guidance on proper posture, ergonomic principles, and body mechanics can help individuals optimize their posture during daily activities and reduce the risk of developing non-specific neck pain.

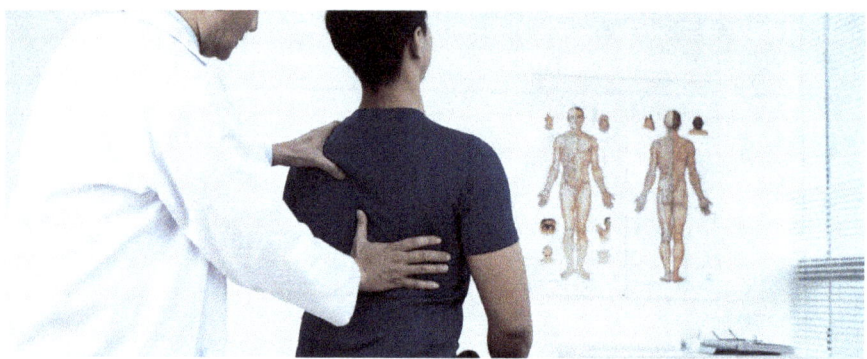

2. Physical Conditioning: Encouraging regular physical activity, including exercises that target neck and shoulder strength, flexibility, and endurance, can help improve physical fitness and reduce the impact of muscular imbalances on neck pain.

3. Stress Management: Offering stress reduction techniques, relaxation strategies, and cognitive-behavioral interventions can help individuals cope with psychosocial stressors and reduce the impact of emotional distress on neck pain.

4. Workplace Interventions: Collaborating with employers to implement ergonomic assessments, modifications to the work environment, and educational programs on healthy work practices can help reduce the impact of occupational factors on neck pain and promote a safe and supportive work environment.

5. Smoking Cessation: Providing resources and support for smoking cessation can help individuals reduce their risk of developing or exacerbating non-specific neck pain and improve overall health outcomes.

In conclusion, non-specific neck pain can be influenced by a variety of contributing factors and risk factors, including poor posture, muscular imbalances, repetitive movements, psychosocial stressors, age, gender, physical fitness, smoking, and occupational factors. Understanding the impact of these factors is essential for healthcare professionals to develop comprehensive treatment plans and preventive strategies for individuals experiencing non-specific neck pain. By addressing physical, psychosocial, and occupational factors, healthcare professionals can help individuals manage non-specific neck pain and reduce the risk of its onset or progression.

### 3. Management and treatment options

Non-specific neck pain is a common musculoskeletal condition that can significantly impact an individual's quality of life and functional abilities. The management and treatment of non-specific neck pain involve a multimodal approach aimed at addressing pain, improving function, and addressing contributing factors. In this article, we will explore various management and treatment options for non-specific neck pain, including conservative measures, interventional therapies, and self-care strategies.

### Conservative Management:

1. <u>Physical Therapy:</u> Physical therapy plays a crucial role in the management of non-specific neck pain. Targeted exercises, manual therapy, and postural education can help improve strength, flexibility, and overall neck health. Physical therapists can develop individualized exercise programs to address muscular imbalances, improve range of motion, and promote proper alignment of the cervical spine. Additionally, ergonomic assessments and modifications may be recommended to optimize the work environment and reduce the impact of occupational factors on neck pain.

2. <u>Pain Medication:</u> Over-the-counter pain medications, such as nonsteroidal anti-inflammatory drugs (NSAIDs) or acetaminophen, may be used to alleviate pain and discomfort

associated with non-specific neck pain. These medications can help reduce inflammation, alleviate muscle tension, and improve the individual's ability to engage in physical therapy and other rehabilitative activities.

3. <u>Heat and Cold Therapy:</u> Applying heat or cold to the affected area can help alleviate muscle stiffness, reduce pain, and promote relaxation. Heat therapy, such as warm compresses or heating pads, can improve blood flow, loosen tight muscles, and enhance tissue flexibility. Cold therapy, such as ice packs or cold compresses, can help reduce inflammation, numb the area, and alleviate acute discomfort.

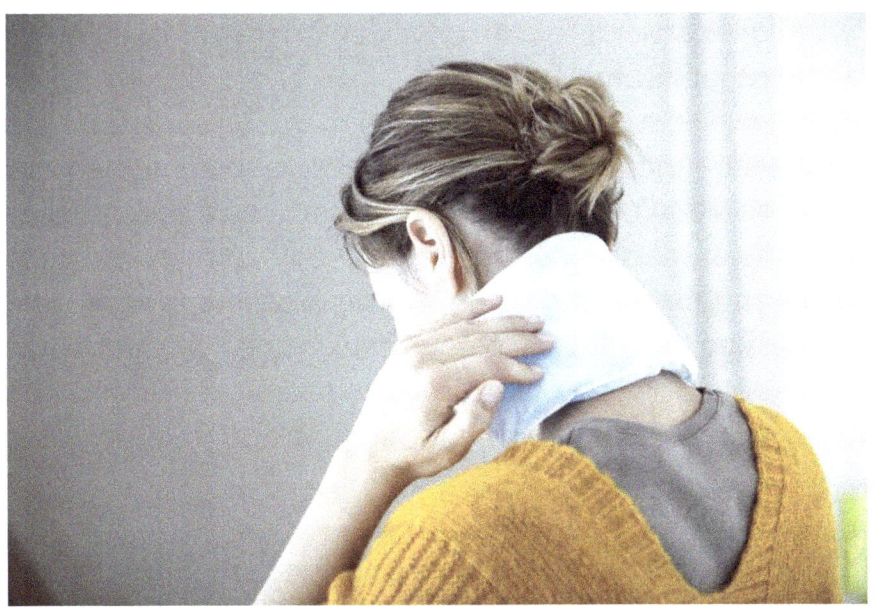

4. <u>Postural Correction:</u> Educating individuals about proper posture and body mechanics is essential

for managing non-specific neck pain. Encouraging ergonomic principles, such as maintaining a neutral spine, adjusting workstation setups, and using supportive seating, can help reduce the strain on the neck and shoulders during daily activities.

## Interventional Therapies:

1. Injections: In some cases, healthcare professionals may recommend injections to alleviate pain and inflammation associated with non-specific neck pain. Corticosteroid injections, such as epidural steroid injections or trigger point injections, can help reduce inflammation, alleviate pain, and improve the individual's ability to participate in physical therapy and other rehabilitative activities.

2. Acupuncture: Acupuncture is a complementary therapy that involves the insertion of thin needles into specific points on the body to alleviate pain and promote healing. Some individuals with non-specific neck pain may find acupuncture beneficial for reducing discomfort, improving muscle relaxation, and enhancing overall well-being.

3. Chiropractic Care: Chiropractic adjustments and manual manipulations may be considered as adjunctive treatments for non-specific neck pain. Chiropractors can perform targeted adjustments

to the cervical spine and surrounding structures to improve joint mobility, reduce muscle tension, and alleviate discomfort.

## Self-Care Strategies:

1. <u>Exercise and Stretching:</u> Engaging in regular exercise and stretching can help improve muscular strength, flexibility, and endurance, reducing the impact of muscular imbalances on non-specific neck pain. Individuals can incorporate gentle neck stretches, shoulder rolls, and upper back exercises into their daily routine to promote mobility and reduce tension.

2. <u>Stress Management:</u> Practicing stress reduction techniques, relaxation strategies, and mindfulness exercises can help individuals cope with psychosocial stressors and reduce the impact of emotional distress on non-specific neck pain. Techniques such as deep breathing, meditation, and progressive muscle relaxation can promote relaxation and improve overall well-being.

3. <u>Ergonomic Modifications:</u> Making ergonomic modifications to the work environment and daily activities can help reduce the impact of occupational factors on non-specific neck pain. Individuals can adjust their workstation setups, use supportive seating, and take regular breaks to minimize the strain on the neck and shoulders

during prolonged sitting or standing.

In conclusion, the management and treatment of non-specific neck pain involve a comprehensive approach that addresses pain, improves function, and targets contributing factors. Conservative measures, such as physical therapy, pain medication, heat and cold therapy, and postural correction, play a key role in the management of non-specific neck pain. Additionally, interventional therapies, including injections, acupuncture, and chiropractic care, may be considered for individuals with persistent or severe symptoms. Self-care strategies, such as exercise and stretching, stress management, and ergonomic modifications, can empower individuals to take an active role in managing their non-specific neck pain and promoting overall well-being. By implementing a multimodal approach that addresses physical, psychosocial, and lifestyle factors, healthcare professionals can help individuals effectively manage non-specific neck pain and improve their quality of life.

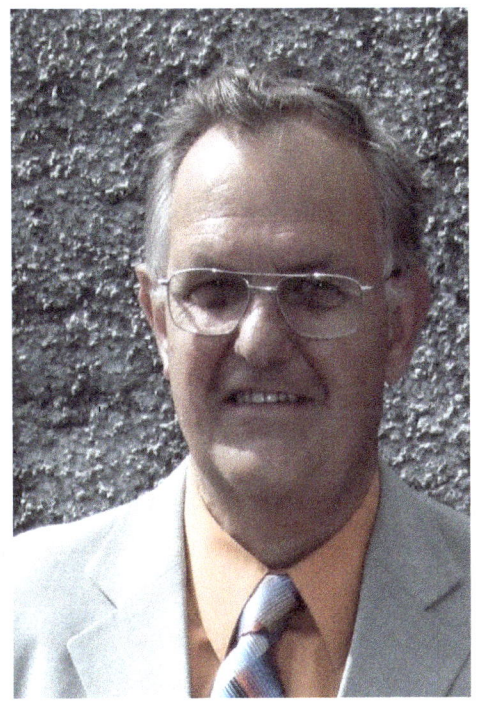

*"It is all very well to say that we use science and mechanical treatment within a holistic framework, but it is too easy for that framework to dissolve in the starry mists of idealism. We all agree in principle that we should treat people and not spines, but then in daily practice we get on with business."*
– Gordon Waddell

# Chapter 4

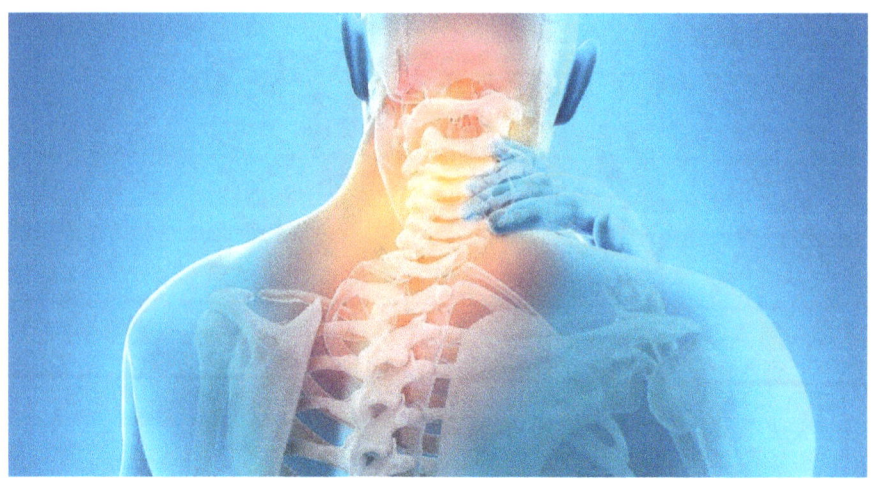

## Specific Neck Conditions

### 1. Cervical spondylosis

Cervical spondylosis, also known as neck arthritis, is a common condition that affects the cervical spine, which is the seven small vertebrae that make up the neck. This condition is caused by the wear and tear of the cartilage and bones in the cervical spine over time. As we age, the discs in our spine can dehydrate and shrink, leading to the development of bone spurs and other degenerative changes. These changes can result in a range of symptoms, including neck pain, stiffness, and in severe cases, numbness or weakness in the arms and legs.

One of the primary symptoms of cervical spondylosis is neck pain. This pain can range from mild to severe and may be exacerbated by certain movements or positions. Many individuals with cervical spondylosis also experience stiffness in the neck, which can make it difficult to turn the head or move the neck freely. In some cases, the degenerative changes in the cervical spine can put pressure on the nerves that extend from the spinal cord to the rest of the body, leading to symptoms such as numbness, tingling, or weakness in the arms and hands.

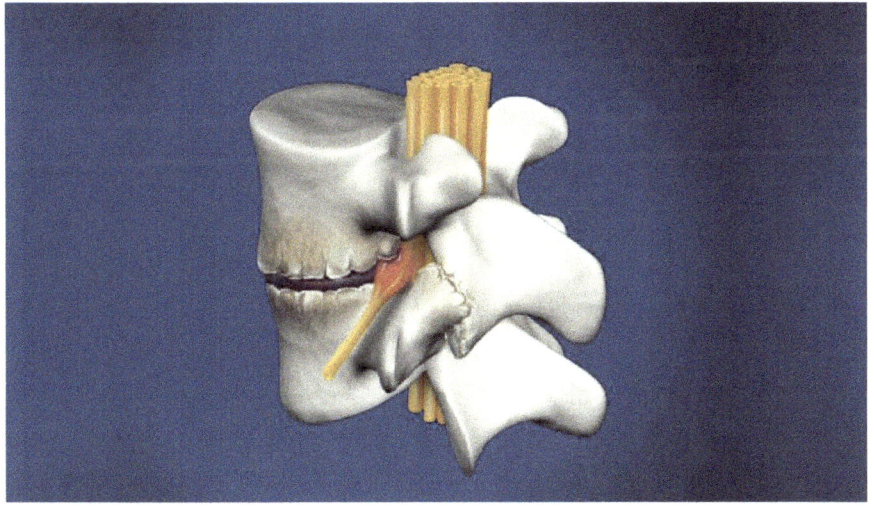

Diagnosing cervical spondylosis typically involves a physical examination, a review of the patient's medical history, and imaging tests such as X-rays, CT scans, or MRI scans. These tests can help to identify the extent of the degenerative changes in the cervical spine and determine the best course of treatment.

Treatment for cervical spondylosis often begins with conservative measures, such as rest, physical therapy, and pain management techniques. Physical therapy can help to improve the strength and flexibility of the neck muscles, while pain management techniques may include the use of over-the-counter or prescription medications, as well as hot or cold therapy. In some cases, corticosteroid injections may be recommended to reduce inflammation and alleviate pain.

For individuals with severe or persistent symptoms, surgical intervention may be necessary. Common surgical procedures for cervical spondylosis include discectomy, in which a portion of a damaged disc is removed, and cervical fusion, in which two or more vertebrae are fused together to stabilize the spine. These procedures can help to relieve pressure on the spinal cord and nerves, and may be performed using minimally invasive techniques to reduce recovery time and minimize the risk of complications.

In addition to medical treatments, individuals with cervical spondylosis can benefit from making lifestyle modifications to manage their symptoms and prevent further degeneration of the cervical spine. This may include maintaining good posture, using ergonomic furniture and equipment, and engaging in regular exercise to strengthen the muscles that support the neck and spine. Weight management and smoking cessation are also important factors in managing cervical spondylosis, as excess weight and smoking can contribute to the degenerative changes in the spine.

Overall, cervical spondylosis is a common and often manageable condition that can cause significant discomfort and limitations in mobility. With proper diagnosis and treatment, individuals with cervical spondylosis can experience relief from their symptoms and improve their quality of life. It is important for individuals experiencing neck pain or other symptoms of cervical spondylosis to seek medical attention in order to receive an accurate diagnosis and develop a personalized treatment plan.

## 2. Cervical radiculopathy

Cervical radiculopathy is a condition characterized by pain and neurological symptoms that result from the compression or irritation of a nerve root in the cervical spine, which is the upper portion of the spinal column located in the neck. This condition can cause a range of symptoms, including neck pain, radiating pain, weakness, numbness, and tingling in the arms and hands. Cervical radiculopathy can be caused by various factors, such as herniated discs, bone spurs, or degenerative changes in the cervical spine.

One of the primary symptoms of cervical radiculopathy is neck pain that radiates into the arm and shoulder. This pain can be sharp or burning in nature and may be exacerbated by certain movements or positions. In addition to pain, individuals with cervical radiculopathy may experience weakness in the muscles of the arm, as well as numbness and tingling in the fingers. These symptoms can significantly impact a person's quality of life, making it difficult to perform everyday tasks and activities.

Diagnosing cervical radiculopathy typically involves a thorough physical examination, a review of the patient's medical history, and imaging tests such as X-rays, CT scans, or MRI scans. These tests can help to identify the location and extent of the nerve compression or irritation, as well as any underlying structural abnormalities in the cervical spine.

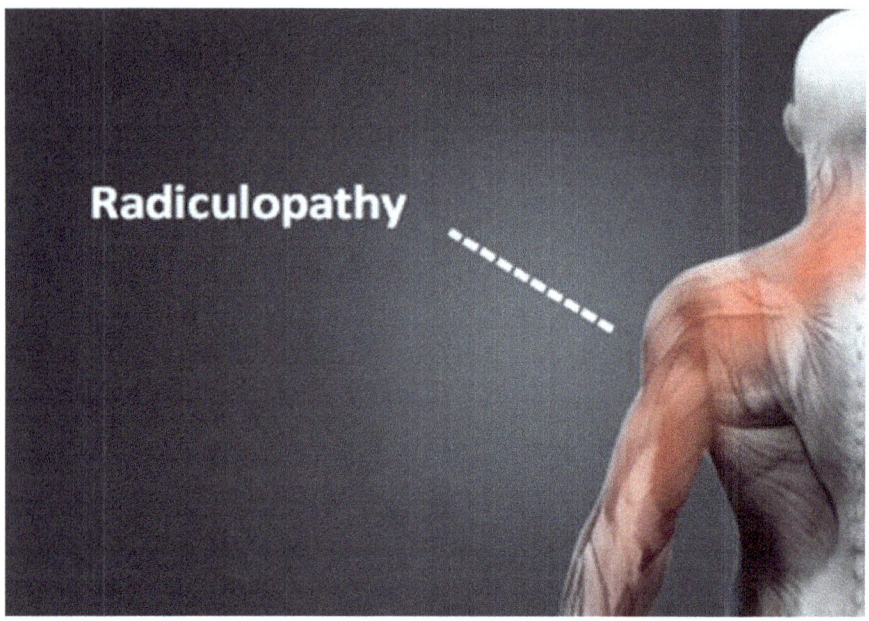

Treatment for cervical radiculopathy often begins with conservative measures aimed at relieving pain and reducing inflammation. This may include rest, physical therapy, and the use of nonsteroidal anti-inflammatory drugs (NSAIDs) to alleviate pain and swelling. Physical therapy can help to improve the strength and flexibility of the neck and shoulder muscles, as well as promote proper posture and body mechanics to reduce strain on the cervical spine.

In some cases, corticosteroid injections may be recommended to reduce inflammation and provide temporary relief from symptoms. These injections are administered directly into the affected area of the spine and can help to alleviate pain and improve mobility. However, it's important to note that the effects of corticosteroid injections are usually temporary and may need to be repeated periodically for ongoing symptom management.

For individuals with severe or persistent symptoms, surgical intervention may be necessary to relieve pressure on the affected nerve root. Common surgical procedures for cervical radiculopathy include discectomy, in which a portion of a herniated disc is removed to alleviate pressure on the nerve, and cervical fusion, in which two or more vertebrae are fused together to stabilize the spine. These procedures can help to alleviate pain and neurological symptoms, and may be performed using minimally invasive techniques to reduce recovery time and minimize the risk of complications.

In addition to medical treatments, individuals with cervical radiculopathy can benefit from making lifestyle modifications to manage their symptoms and prevent further nerve compression. This may include maintaining good posture, using ergonomic furniture and equipment, and engaging in regular exercise to strengthen the muscles that support the neck and spine. Weight management and smoking cessation are also important factors in managing cervical radiculopathy, as excess weight and smoking can contribute to the degenerative changes in the spine.

Overall, cervical radiculopathy is a challenging condition that can cause significant discomfort and limitations in mobility. With proper diagnosis and treatment, individuals with cervical radiculopathy can experience relief from their symptoms and improve their quality of life. It is important for individuals experiencing neck pain, weakness, or neurological symptoms to seek medical attention in order to receive an accurate diagnosis and develop a personalized treatment plan.

## 3. Whiplash-associated disorders and other specific conditions

Whiplash-associated disorders (WAD) and other specific conditions in neck pain encompass a range of injuries and medical conditions that affect the neck and surrounding structures. These conditions can result from various causes, including trauma, degenerative changes, and underlying medical conditions. Understanding these specific conditions is crucial for accurate diagnosis and effective management of neck pain.

Whiplash-associated disorders (WAD) are a group of symptoms that occur following a sudden acceleration-deceleration force, which causes the neck to move beyond its normal range of motion. This type of injury is commonly associated with motor vehicle accidents, but it can also result from sports-related injuries, falls, or physical assaults. The primary symptoms of WAD include neck pain, stiffness, headaches, and in some cases, neurological symptoms such as numbness, tingling, or weakness in the arms and hands.

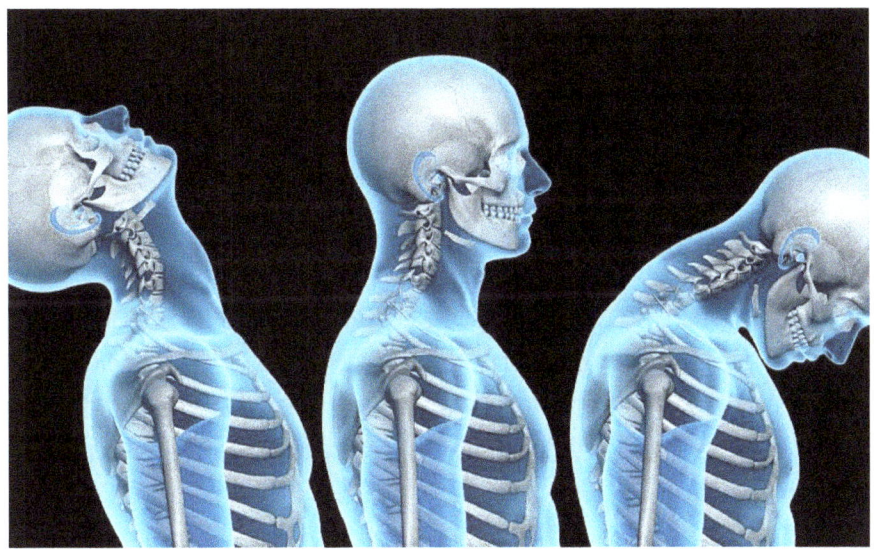

Diagnosing WAD typically involves a thorough physical examination, a review of the patient's medical history, and imaging tests such as X-rays, CT scans, or MRI scans. These tests can help to identify any structural abnormalities in the cervical spine, as well as assess the extent of soft tissue damage. It's important to note that the severity of symptoms in WAD can vary widely, and some individuals may experience persistent pain and disability following the initial injury.

Treatment for WAD often begins with conservative measures aimed at relieving pain and promoting healing of the injured tissues. This may include rest, physical therapy, and the use of pain medications or muscle relaxants to alleviate discomfort. Physical therapy plays a crucial role in WAD recovery by focusing on restoring range of motion, strengthening the neck muscles, and improving posture. Additionally, modalities such as heat, ice, and ultrasound may be used to reduce pain and inflammation.

In some cases, corticosteroid injections may be recommended to reduce inflammation and provide temporary relief from symptoms. These injections are administered directly into the affected area of the spine and can help to alleviate pain and improve mobility. However, it's important to note that the effects of corticosteroid injections are usually temporary and may need to be repeated periodically for ongoing symptom management.

For individuals with persistent or severe symptoms, more advanced interventions such as nerve blocks or radiofrequency ablation may be considered to target specific nerves and provide longer-lasting pain relief. These procedures are typically performed by pain management specialists and can be effective in managing chronic neck pain associated with WAD.

In addition to WAD, there are other specific conditions that can cause neck pain and related symptoms. Conditions such as cervical dystonia, a neurological movement disorder characterized by involuntary muscle contractions in the neck, and cervical spinal stenosis, a narrowing of the spinal canal in the neck, can also contribute to neck pain and related symptoms. These conditions require specialized evaluation and management by healthcare professionals with expertise in neurology and spinal disorders.

Overall, the management of whiplash-associated disorders and other specific conditions in neck pain requires a comprehensive approach that addresses the underlying causes of symptoms and aims to improve function and quality of life. It is essential for individuals experiencing neck pain, stiffness, or neurological symptoms to seek medical attention in order to receive an accurate diagnosis and develop a personalized treatment plan tailored to their specific needs. By understanding the complexities of these conditions, healthcare providers can offer effective interventions that help individuals recover from neck pain and regain optimal neck function.

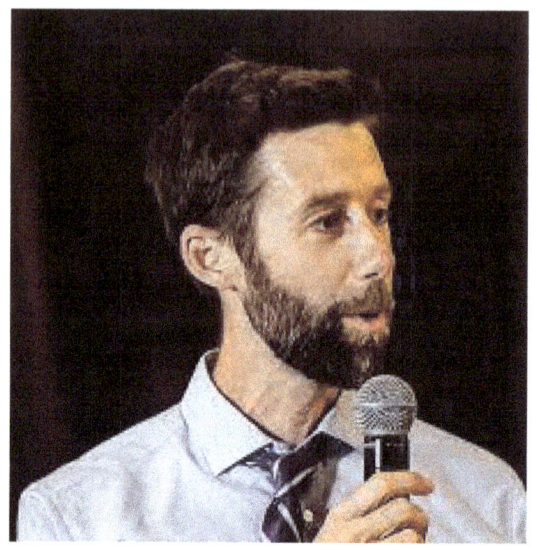

*"When neck pain suddenly shows up, we are tempted to blame it on the last minor stressor that affected it, such as a soft bed in a hotel. This is like blaming your bankruptcy on the last latte you bought before your account finally went into the red."*

– Todd Hargrove

# Chapter 5

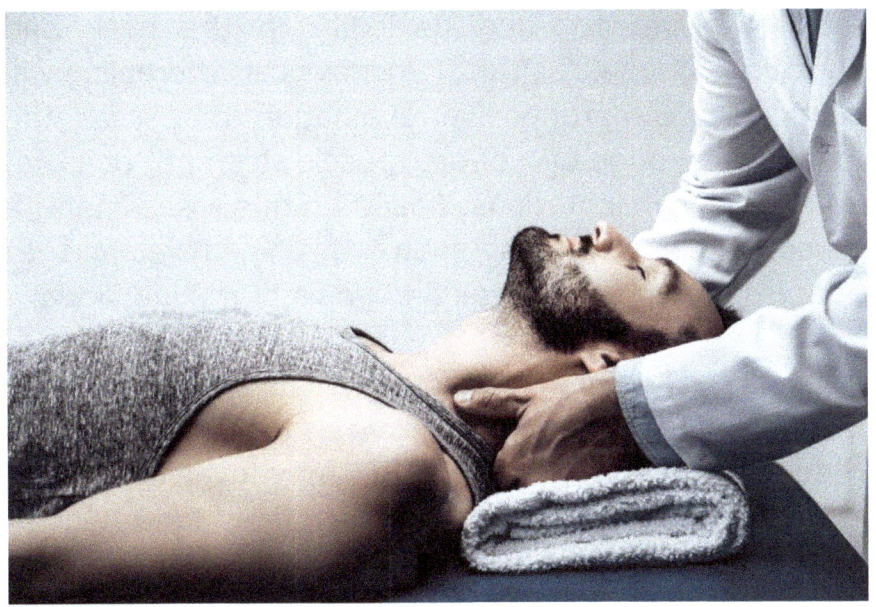

## Conservative Treatment Approaches

### 1. Physical therapy and exercise

Conservative treatment approaches, such as physical therapy and exercise, play a crucial role in managing neck pain and promoting recovery. These interventions are often recommended as first-line treatments for individuals with acute or chronic neck pain, as they can help to alleviate symptoms, improve function, and prevent future episodes of pain. Understanding the principles and benefits of physical therapy and exercise in the management of neck pain is essential for both healthcare providers and individuals seeking relief from this common condition.

Physical therapy is a cornerstone of conservative treatment for neck pain, as it focuses on restoring mobility, strength, and flexibility in the neck and surrounding musculature. A physical therapist will conduct a comprehensive evaluation to assess the individual's range of motion, muscle strength, posture, and functional limitations. Based on this assessment, a personalized treatment plan will be developed to address the specific needs and goals of the individual.

One of the primary goals of physical therapy in neck pain management is to improve range of motion and reduce stiffness in the neck. This may involve targeted stretching exercises that aim to lengthen tight muscles and improve flexibility in the cervical spine. Gentle, controlled movements are used to gradually increase the range of motion without causing further discomfort or strain.

In addition to addressing range of motion, physical therapy also focuses on strengthening the muscles that support the neck and upper back. Weakness in these muscles can contribute to poor posture and increased stress on the cervical spine, leading to pain and dysfunction. Through targeted strengthening exercises, individuals can improve the stability and endurance of these muscles, which can help to alleviate neck pain and reduce the risk of future injuries.

Posture correction is another important component of physical therapy for neck pain. Poor posture can place excessive strain on the neck and upper back, leading to muscle imbalances and increased stress on the spinal structures. A physical therapist can provide guidance on proper body mechanics and ergonomics, as well as prescribe exercises and techniques to promote optimal posture during daily activities.

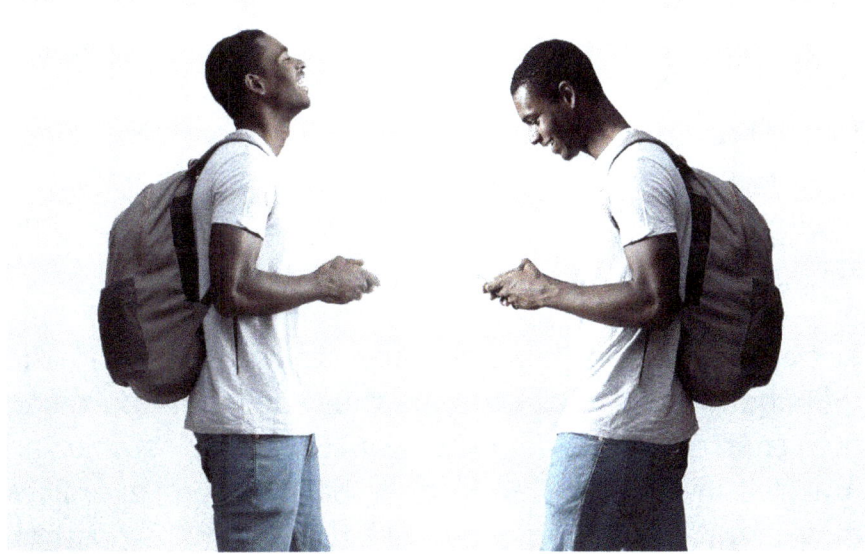

Furthermore, physical therapy may incorporate modalities such as heat, ice, ultrasound, and electrical stimulation to reduce pain and inflammation in the neck. These modalities can provide temporary relief from discomfort and help to facilitate the healing process, particularly in the acute stages of neck pain.

Exercise is an integral component of conservative treatment for neck pain, as it complements the goals of physical therapy and promotes overall musculoskeletal health. Aerobic exercise, such as walking, cycling, or swimming, can help to improve cardiovascular fitness and promote circulation, which can support the healing process and reduce stiffness in the neck.

In addition to aerobic exercise, specific neck exercises can target the muscles and structures that are commonly affected by neck pain. These exercises may include neck stretches, isometric exercises, and dynamic movements that aim to improve mobility, strength, and coordination in the cervical spine. Individuals are typically instructed to perform these exercises under the guidance of a physical therapist or healthcare provider to ensure proper technique and safety.

Neck stabilization exercises are also important in the management of neck pain, as they focus on improving the control and endurance of the deep stabilizing muscles in the neck and upper back. These exercises may involve gentle movements that promote postural awareness and core stability, which can help to reduce strain on the cervical spine and improve overall function.

Moreover, individuals with neck pain can benefit from incorporating relaxation techniques and stress management strategies into their exercise routine. Stress and tension can exacerbate neck pain and contribute to muscle tightness, so techniques such as deep breathing, meditation, and progressive muscle relaxation can help to alleviate these symptoms and promote a sense of well-being.

It's important to note that the effectiveness of physical therapy and exercise in the management of neck pain is supported by a growing body of evidence. Research has shown that these interventions can lead to improvements in pain, function, and quality of life for individuals with acute and chronic neck pain, and are associated with a lower risk of recurrent symptoms compared to passive treatments alone.

In conclusion, physical therapy and exercise are essential components of conservative treatment approaches in neck pain management. These interventions aim to improve mobility, strength, and function in the neck and surrounding musculature, and can help to alleviate symptoms, prevent future episodes of pain, and promote overall musculoskeletal health. By incorporating physical therapy and exercise into a comprehensive treatment plan, individuals with neck pain can experience meaningful improvements in their condition and regain optimal neck function.

## 2. Pain management techniques

Pain management techniques play a crucial role in the comprehensive treatment of neck pain, aiming to alleviate discomfort, improve function, and enhance the overall quality of life for individuals affected by this common condition. Understanding the principles and benefits of pain management techniques in the context of neck pain is essential for both healthcare providers and individuals seeking relief from this often debilitating issue.

One of the primary goals of pain management in neck pain is to reduce discomfort and improve the individual's ability to perform daily activities. This can be achieved through a combination of pharmacological and non-pharmacological interventions, tailored to the specific needs and preferences of the individual.

Pharmacological interventions for neck pain management often include the use of nonsteroidal anti-inflammatory drugs (NSAIDs), such as ibuprofen or naproxen, to reduce pain and inflammation in the affected area. These medications can be effective in alleviating mild to moderate neck pain and are often used as a first-line treatment for acute episodes of discomfort. However, it's important to use NSAIDs cautiously, as long-term or excessive use can lead to gastrointestinal issues and other potential side effects.

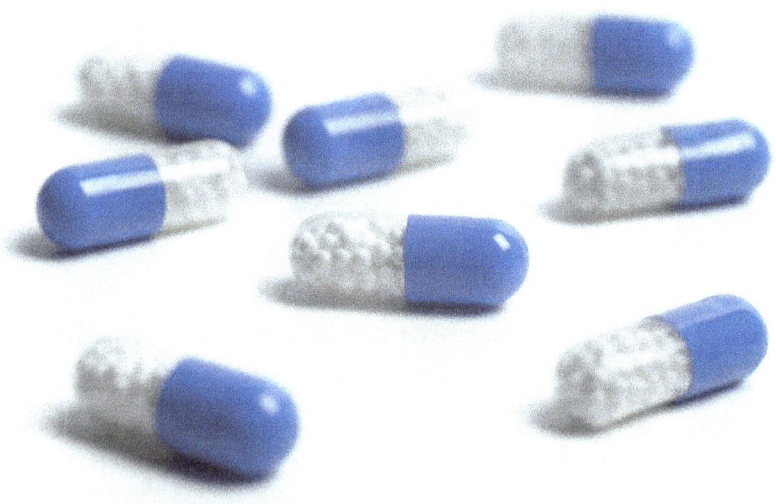

In addition to NSAIDs, muscle relaxants may be prescribed to alleviate muscle spasms and tension in the neck and upper back. These medications can help to reduce discomfort and improve mobility, particularly in cases where muscle tightness contributes to the individual's symptoms.

For individuals with more severe or persistent neck pain, opioid medications may be considered for short-term use under close supervision by a healthcare provider. Opioids can provide effective pain relief, but their use is associated with a risk of tolerance, dependence, and potential adverse effects. Therefore, they are typically reserved for cases where other treatments have been ineffective, and their use is carefully monitored to minimize the risk of misuse or dependency.

In addition to pharmacological interventions, non-pharmacological pain management techniques are an essential component of neck pain treatment. Physical therapy, for example, plays a crucial role in pain management by addressing muscle imbalances, improving posture, and promoting optimal function in the neck and surrounding musculature. Through targeted exercises, manual therapy, and modalities such as heat, ice, and electrical stimulation, physical therapists can help individuals alleviate discomfort and improve their overall musculoskeletal health.

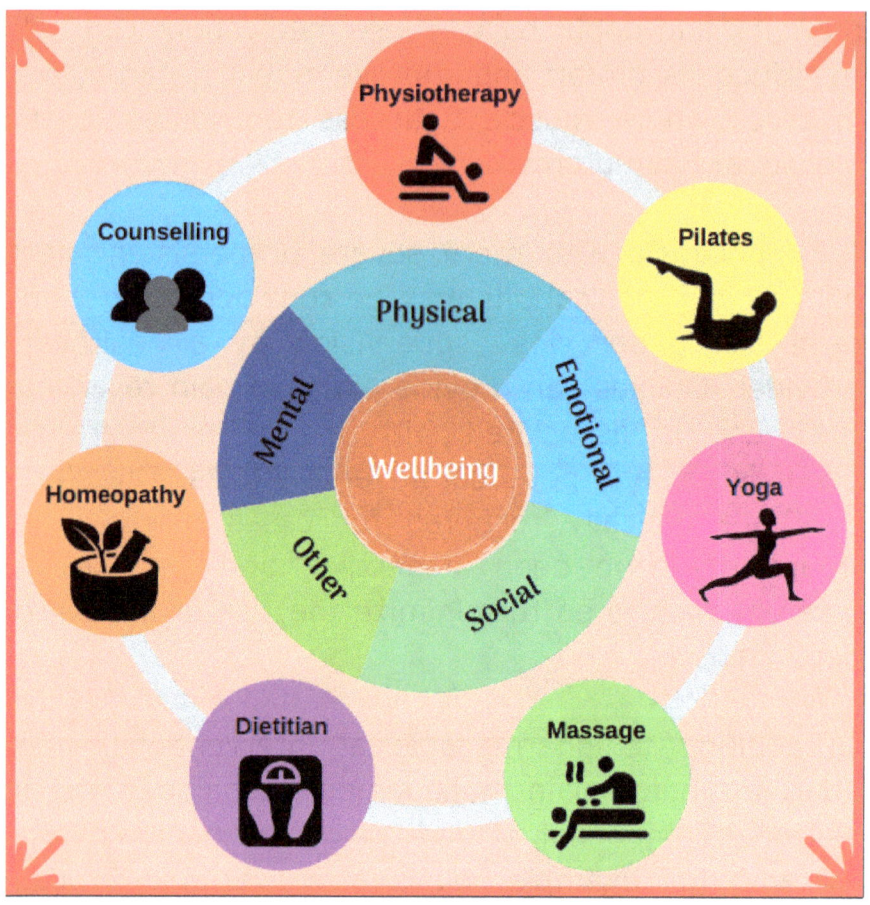

Furthermore, complementary and alternative therapies, such as acupuncture, chiropractic care, and massage therapy, can be valuable additions to a comprehensive pain management plan for neck pain. These therapies aim to reduce pain, improve mobility, and promote relaxation, and are often well-received by individuals seeking natural and holistic approaches to pain relief.

Psychological interventions are also important in the management of neck pain, as they can help individuals cope with the emotional and psychological impact of chronic discomfort. Cognitive-behavioral therapy (CBT), for example, focuses on changing negative thought patterns and behaviors related to pain, and has been shown to be effective in improving pain coping skills and overall well-being.

Moreover, relaxation techniques, such as deep breathing, meditation, and progressive muscle relaxation, can help individuals manage stress and tension, which can exacerbate neck pain and contribute to muscle tightness. By incorporating these techniques into their daily routine, individuals can experience relief from discomfort and improve their overall quality of life.

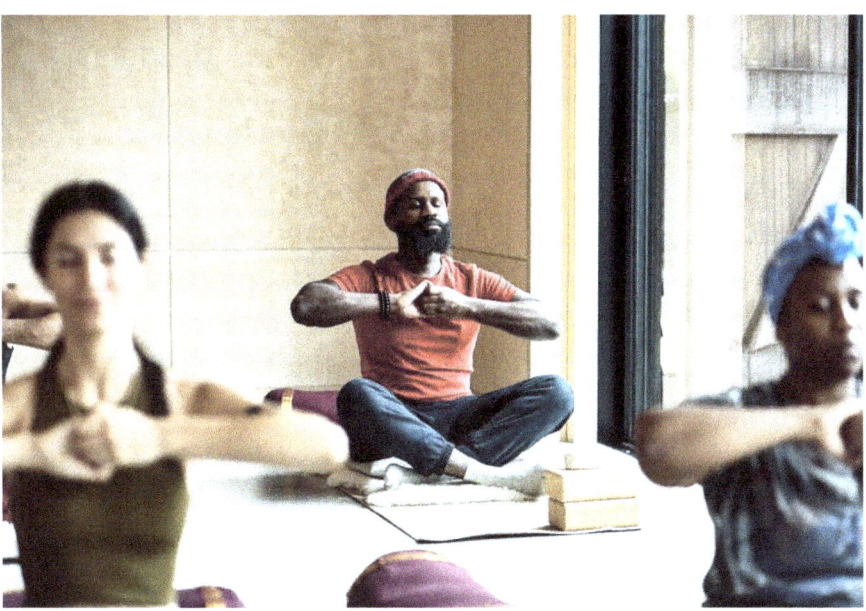

In some cases, interventional pain management procedures may be considered for individuals with severe or refractory neck pain. These procedures, which are typically performed by pain management specialists, aim to target specific nerves or structures in the cervical spine to alleviate pain and improve function. Common interventional procedures for neck pain include epidural steroid injections, facet joint injections, and radiofrequency ablation, which can provide targeted pain relief and may be effective in managing chronic discomfort.

It's important to note that the effectiveness of pain management techniques in neck pain is supported by a growing body of evidence. Research has shown that a multimodal approach to pain management, which combines pharmacological, non-pharmacological, and interventional interventions, can lead to improvements in pain, function, and quality of life for individuals with acute and chronic neck pain.

In conclusion, pain management techniques are essential components of the comprehensive treatment of neck pain, aiming to alleviate discomfort, improve function, and enhance the overall quality of life for affected individuals. By incorporating a combination of pharmacological and non-pharmacological interventions, tailored to the specific needs and preferences of the individual, healthcare providers can offer effective pain relief and support individuals in their journey towards recovery and optimal neck function.

## 3. Lifestyle modifications and ergonomic considerations

Lifestyle modifications and ergonomic considerations play a crucial role in the management of neck pain, aiming to reduce discomfort, prevent further injury, and promote optimal musculoskeletal health. Understanding the principles and benefits of lifestyle modifications and ergonomic considerations in the context of neck pain is essential for both healthcare providers and individuals seeking relief from this common and often debilitating condition.

One of the primary goals of lifestyle modifications in neck pain management is to identify and address factors that contribute to discomfort and dysfunction in daily life. This may include addressing poor posture, reducing sedentary behavior, and promoting healthy lifestyle habits that support optimal musculoskeletal health.

Posture correction is a key component of lifestyle modifications for neck pain. Poor posture, such as slouching or hunching over, can place excessive strain on the neck and upper back, leading to muscle imbalances and increased stress on the spinal structures. Individuals with neck pain can benefit from ergonomic assessments to identify and address poor posture in various settings, such as at work, during leisure activities, and while performing household tasks.

Ergonomic considerations are essential in the management of neck pain, as they aim to optimize the individual's physical environment to reduce strain on the neck and upper back. This may include adjusting the height and positioning of workstations, using supportive seating with proper lumbar support, and incorporating ergonomic tools and accessories, such as adjustable desks and chairs, to promote neutral body positioning and reduce the risk of musculoskeletal discomfort.

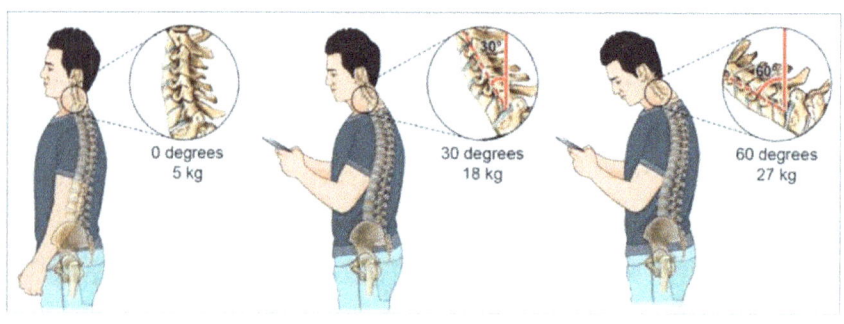

In addition to posture correction and ergonomic considerations, individuals with neck pain can benefit from incorporating regular movement and physical activity into their daily routine. Prolonged periods of sitting or sedentary behavior can contribute to muscle stiffness and tension in the neck and upper back, exacerbating discomfort and reducing overall musculoskeletal health. By incorporating regular breaks, stretching exercises, and movement into their daily activities, individuals can reduce the risk of developing or exacerbating neck pain.

Furthermore, maintaining a healthy weight and engaging in regular exercise can support optimal musculoskeletal health and reduce the risk of developing or exacerbating neck pain. Excess weight can place additional strain on the neck and upper back, leading to muscle imbalances and increased stress on the spinal structures. By adopting a healthy diet and engaging in regular physical activity, individuals can reduce the risk of musculoskeletal discomfort and promote overall well-being.

Smoking cessation is another important lifestyle modification for individuals with neck pain. Smoking has been associated with an increased risk of developing degenerative changes in the spine, such as disc degeneration and osteoarthritis, which can contribute to neck pain and dysfunction. By quitting smoking, individuals can reduce the risk of developing or exacerbating neck pain and support optimal musculoskeletal health.

In addition to lifestyle modifications, ergonomic considerations are essential in the management of neck pain, as they aim to optimize the individual's physical environment to reduce strain on the neck and upper back. This may include adjusting the height and positioning of workstations, using supportive seating with proper lumbar support, and incorporating ergonomic tools and accessories, such as adjustable desks and chairs, to promote neutral body positioning and reduce the risk of musculoskeletal discomfort.

It's important to note that the effectiveness of lifestyle modifications and ergonomic considerations in neck pain management is supported by a growing body of evidence. Research has shown that these interventions can lead to improvements in posture, musculoskeletal health, and overall well-being for individuals with acute and chronic neck pain, and are associated with a lower risk of recurrent symptoms compared to passive treatments alone.

In conclusion, lifestyle modifications and ergonomic considerations are essential components of the comprehensive management of neck pain, aiming to reduce discomfort, prevent further injury, and promote optimal musculoskeletal health. By addressing factors such as posture, movement, weight management, and stress, individuals can reduce the risk of developing or exacerbating neck pain and support their journey towards recovery and optimal neck function.

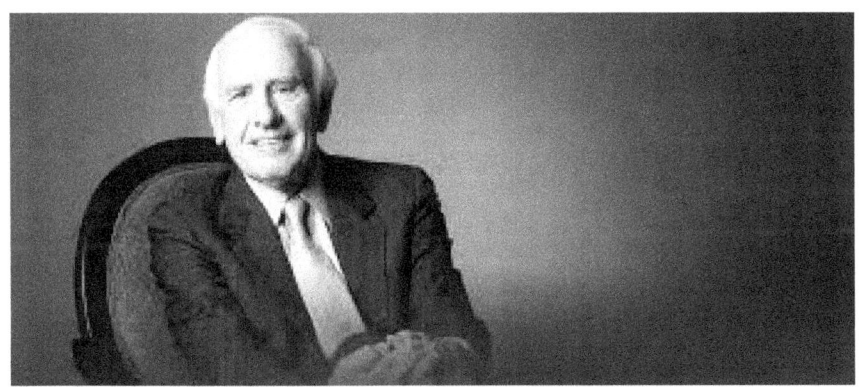

**"Take care of your body. It's the only place you have to live."**

– Jim Rohn

# Chapter 6

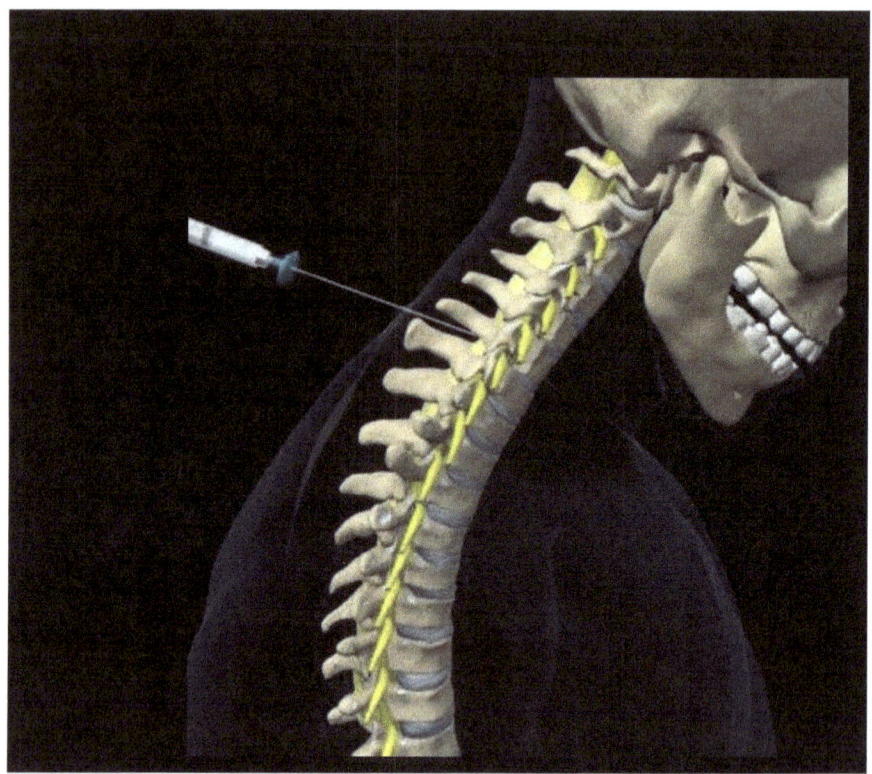

## Interventional and Surgical Options

### 1. Epidural steroid injections

Interventional and surgical options play a crucial role in the management of neck pain, particularly for individuals with severe or refractory symptoms that have not responded to conservative treatments. Among the interventional options, epidural steroid injections are a commonly utilized procedure aimed at providing targeted pain relief and reducing inflammation in the cervical spine. Understanding the principles, benefits, and considerations of epidural steroid injections in the context of neck pain is essential for both healthcare providers and individuals seeking relief from this often debilitating condition.

Epidural steroid injections involve the administration of a corticosteroid medication, often combined with a local anesthetic, into the epidural space of the cervical spine. The epidural space is the area surrounding the dura, which contains the spinal cord and nerve roots. By delivering medication directly into this space, epidural steroid injections can target inflamed or compressed nerves, reduce pain, and improve function in individuals with neck pain.

The primary goal of epidural steroid injections in neck pain management is to reduce inflammation and alleviate pain associated with conditions such as cervical radiculopathy, herniated discs, spinal stenosis, and other spinal disorders. These injections can provide targeted relief by delivering medication directly to the affected area, thereby minimizing systemic side effects and maximizing the therapeutic effect on the inflamed or compressed nerves.

The procedure for epidural steroid injections typically involves the following steps:

1. Pre-procedure Evaluation: Before the injection, the healthcare provider will conduct a thorough evaluation of the individual's medical history, symptoms, and imaging studies to confirm the diagnosis and identify the specific area of nerve

compression or inflammation.

2. <u>Informed Consent:</u> The healthcare provider will discuss the risks, benefits, and potential outcomes of the procedure with the individual, and obtain informed consent prior to the injection.

3. <u>Injection Technique:</u> The individual will be positioned on an examination table, and the skin overlying the injection site will be cleansed and anesthetized. Using fluoroscopic guidance or ultrasound, the healthcare provider will carefully insert a needle into the epidural space and confirm its placement using contrast dye.

4. <u>Medication Delivery</u>: Once the needle is properly positioned, the corticosteroid medication, often combined with a local anesthetic, is injected into the epidural space. The medication spreads around the inflamed or compressed nerves, reducing inflammation and providing pain relief.

5. <u>Post-procedure Monitoring</u>: After the injection, the individual will be monitored for a short period to ensure there are no immediate complications, and then discharged with instructions for post-procedure care.

The effects of epidural steroid injections can vary among individuals, but many experience a reduction in pain and inflammation within a few days following the procedure. It's important to note that while these injections can provide significant relief, the effects are often temporary and may need to be repeated periodically for ongoing symptom management.

## Cervical Epidural Steroid Injection

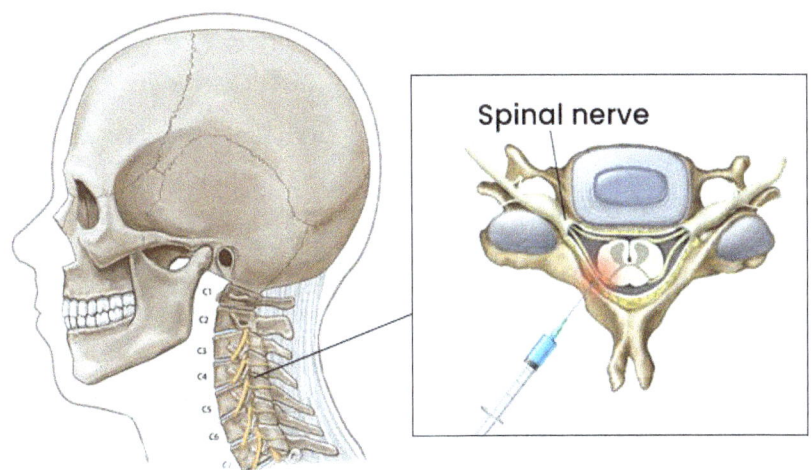

In addition to providing pain relief, epidural steroid injections can also serve a diagnostic purpose. By observing the individual's response to the injection, healthcare providers can gain valuable information about the specific source of pain and the potential effectiveness of other treatments, including surgical options, if necessary.

While epidural steroid injections are generally considered safe, there are potential risks and considerations that individuals should be aware of. These may include temporary increases in pain, infection at the injection site, allergic reactions to the medication, and rare but serious complications such as nerve damage or spinal cord injury. Therefore, it's essential for individuals to discuss the potential risks and benefits of the procedure with their healthcare provider and make an informed decision based on their specific condition and medical history.

In conclusion, epidural steroid injections are a valuable interventional option in the management of neck pain, particularly for individuals with nerve-related symptoms and inflammation in the cervical spine. By delivering targeted pain relief and reducing inflammation, these injections can help individuals regain function and improve their quality of life. However, it's important for individuals to work closely with their healthcare provider to determine if epidural steroid injections are an appropriate option for their specific condition and to weigh the potential risks and benefits before proceeding with the procedure.

## 2. Minimally invasive procedures

Minimally invasive procedures have revolutionized the field of back pain management, offering effective treatment options with reduced recovery times, less post-operative pain, and lower risk of complications compared to traditional open surgeries. These procedures utilize advanced techniques and technologies to address a wide range of spinal conditions, providing targeted relief for individuals suffering from back pain. Understanding the principles, benefits, and considerations of minimally invasive procedures in the context of neck pain is essential for both healthcare providers and individuals seeking relief from this often debilitating condition.

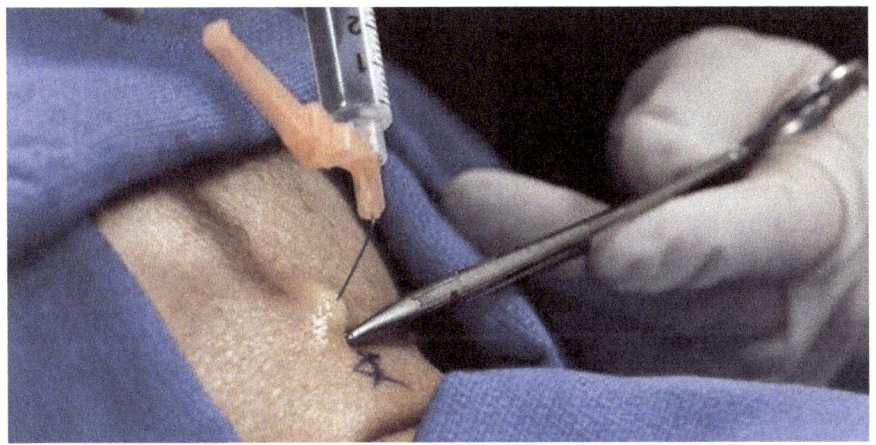

One of the key advantages of minimally invasive procedures in neck pain management is the ability to target specific sources of pain and pathology with minimal disruption to surrounding tissues. These procedures are often performed using small incisions, specialized instruments, and advanced imaging guidance, allowing healthcare providers to access the affected area of the spine with precision and accuracy. By minimizing tissue trauma and preserving healthy structures, minimally invasive procedures can lead to faster recovery, reduced post-operative pain, and improved functional outcomes for individuals with back pain.

There are several minimally invasive procedures commonly used in the management of back pain, each tailored to address specific spinal conditions and symptoms. Some of the most widely utilized minimally invasive procedures include:

1. Discectomy: A discectomy is a minimally invasive procedure performed to remove a portion of a herniated or bulging disc that is pressing on a nerve root or the spinal cord. This procedure can alleviate nerve compression, reduce pain, and improve mobility in individuals with symptoms such as sciatica or radiculopathy. Minimally invasive discectomy techniques often involve the use of a small incision, specialized instruments, and microscopic or endoscopic visualization to access the affected disc and remove the herniated portion, while preserving as much of the healthy disc tissue as possible.

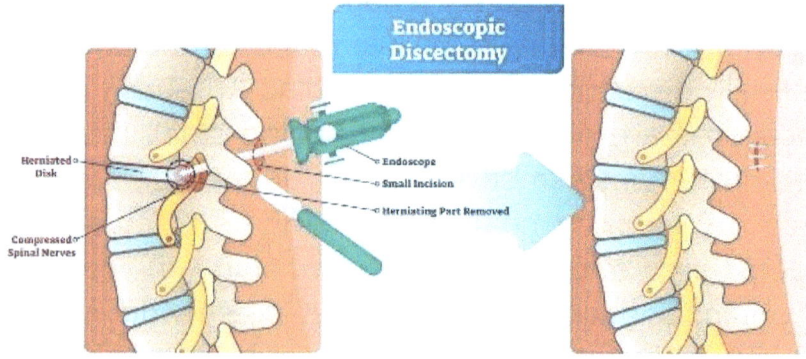

2. Laminectomy: A laminectomy, also known as decompression surgery, is a minimally invasive procedure aimed at relieving pressure on the spinal cord or nerve roots by removing a portion of the lamina, the bony arch of the vertebra. This procedure is commonly performed to address

spinal stenosis, a condition characterized by the narrowing of the spinal canal, which can lead to compression of the spinal cord and nerves. Minimally invasive laminectomy techniques utilize small incisions, specialized tools, and advanced imaging to access the affected area of the spine and remove the necessary bone and tissue, while minimizing disruption to surrounding structures.

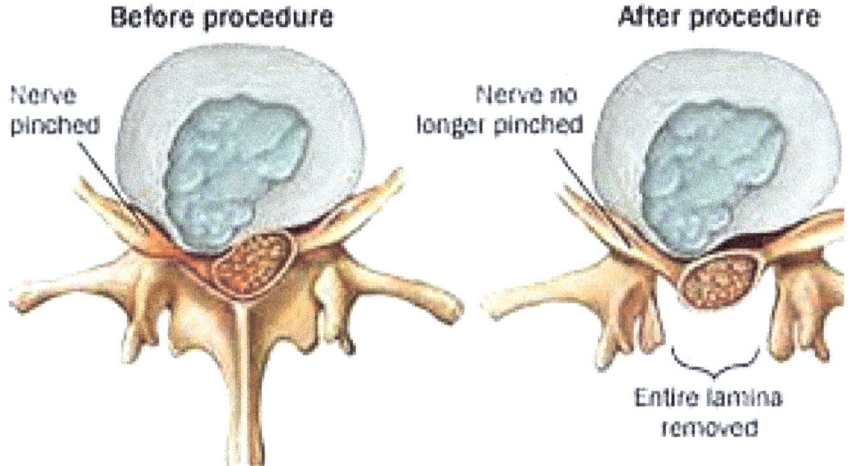

3. Spinal Fusion: Minimally invasive spinal fusion is a procedure performed to stabilize the spine and reduce pain by fusing two or more vertebrae together. This procedure is often used to address conditions such as degenerative disc disease, spondylolisthesis, or spinal instability. Minimally invasive spinal fusion techniques involve the use of small incisions, specialized implants, and advanced imaging guidance to access the spine and place bone graft material or implants to promote fusion, while minimizing disruption to

the surrounding muscles and tissues.

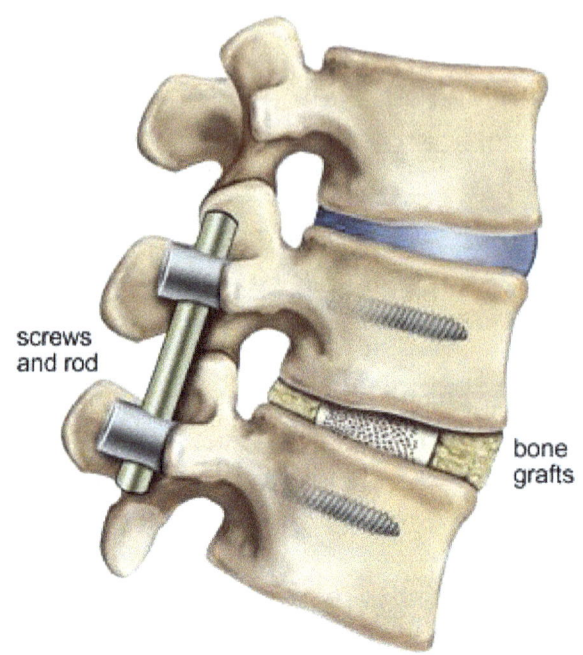

screws
and rod

bone
grafts

4. <u>Vertebroplasty and Kyphoplasty</u>: Vertebroplasty and kyphoplasty are minimally invasive procedures used to treat vertebral compression fractures, which can cause severe back pain and spinal deformity. During vertebroplasty, bone cement is injected into the fractured vertebra to stabilize the bone and alleviate pain. Kyphoplasty involves the use of a balloon-like device to create space in the fractured vertebra before injecting the bone cement, aiming to restore vertebral height and alignment. These procedures are performed using small incisions and specialized instruments, providing rapid pain relief and improved spinal stability for individuals with

vertebral compression fractures.

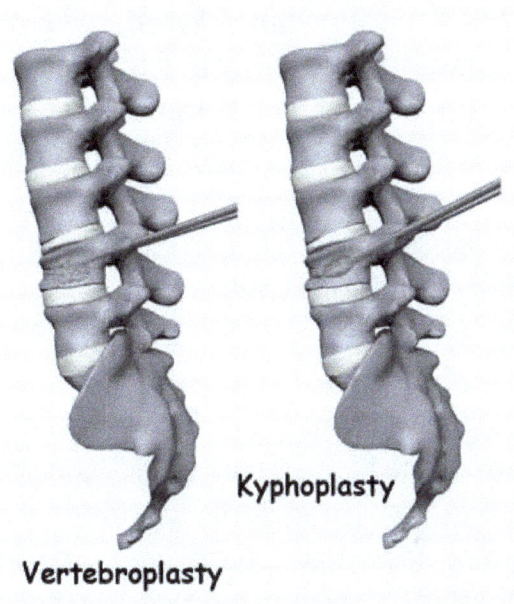

**Kyphoplasty**

**Vertebroplasty**

5. <u>Minimally Invasive Lumbar Decompression (MILD)</u>: MILD is a minimally invasive procedure designed to address lumbar spinal stenosis, a common cause of lower back and leg pain. This procedure involves the use of specialized tools and imaging guidance to remove overgrown bone and tissue, relieving pressure on the spinal nerves and restoring mobility. MILD is performed through small incisions, allowing for a quicker recovery and reduced risk of complications compared to traditional open surgeries.

It's important to note that while minimally invasive procedures offer significant benefits for individuals with back pain, they are not suitable for all spinal conditions or all patients. Healthcare providers carefully evaluate each individual's medical history, symptoms, and diagnostic imaging to determine the most appropriate treatment approach. Additionally, individuals considering minimally invasive procedures should discuss the potential risks, benefits, and expected outcomes with their healthcare provider to make an informed decision about their care.

In conclusion, minimally invasive procedures have transformed the landscape of back pain management, offering effective treatment options with reduced recovery times, less post-operative pain, and lower risk of complications compared to traditional open surgeries. These procedures provide targeted relief for a wide range of spinal conditions, allowing individuals to regain function and improve their quality of life. By understanding the principles, benefits, and considerations of minimally invasive procedures, healthcare providers and individuals can work together to develop personalized treatment plans that address the specific needs and goals of each patient, ultimately leading to improved outcomes and enhanced well-being.

### 3. Surgical interventions for specific conditions

Surgical interventions for specific conditions in neck pain play a crucial role in the management of severe or refractory symptoms that have not responded to conservative treatments. These surgical procedures are designed to address underlying structural issues in the cervical spine, alleviate nerve compression, stabilize the spine, and improve overall function and quality of life for individuals with debilitating neck pain. Understanding the specific conditions that may require surgical intervention, as well as the available surgical options, is essential for healthcare providers and individuals considering surgical treatment for neck pain.

One of the common conditions that may necessitate surgical intervention is cervical radiculopathy, which results from the compression or irritation of a nerve root in the cervical spine. This condition can cause pain, weakness, numbness, and tingling that radiates into the arms and hands. Surgical options for cervical radiculopathy may include discectomy, in which a portion of a herniated disc is removed to alleviate pressure on the nerve, and cervical fusion, in which two or more vertebrae are fused together to stabilize the spine and reduce nerve compression. These surgical procedures aim to address the underlying cause of nerve compression and provide lasting relief from symptoms.

Another specific condition that may require surgical intervention is cervical spondylosis, also known as neck arthritis. This condition results from the wear and tear of the cervical spine over time, leading to the development of bone spurs, herniated discs, and other structural changes that can cause neck pain, stiffness, and neurological symptoms. Surgical options for cervical spondylosis may include decompressive laminectomy, in which the lamina and other structures causing compression are removed to alleviate pressure on the spinal cord and nerves, and cervical fusion to stabilize the affected segments of the spine.

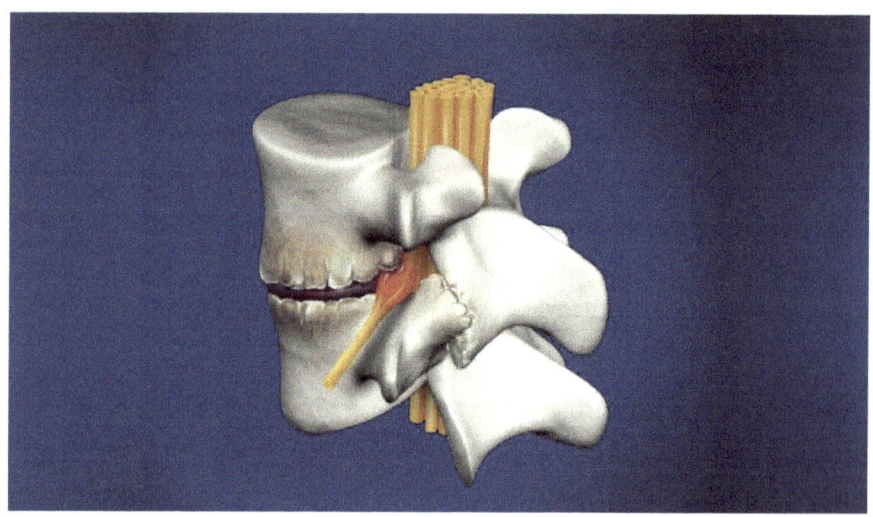

In addition to cervical radiculopathy and cervical spondylosis, other specific conditions such as cervical disc herniation, spinal stenosis, and cervical myelopathy may also require surgical intervention to address severe or progressive symptoms. Surgical procedures for cervical disc herniation may involve discectomy to remove the herniated portion of the disc, while spinal stenosis may be treated with decompressive laminectomy or laminoplasty to alleviate pressure on the spinal cord and nerves. Cervical myelopathy, a condition characterized by compression of the spinal cord, may require surgical decompression and stabilization to prevent further neurological deterioration.

It's important to note that surgical interventions for specific conditions in neck pain are typically considered after conservative treatments have been exhausted and when symptoms significantly impact an individual's quality of life and function. Healthcare providers carefully evaluate each individual's medical history, diagnostic imaging, and response to conservative treatments to determine the most appropriate surgical approach. Additionally, individuals considering surgical intervention for neck pain should discuss the potential risks, benefits, and expected outcomes with their healthcare provider to make an informed decision about their care.

Advancements in surgical techniques and technology have led to the development of minimally invasive surgical approaches for specific conditions in neck pain. Minimally invasive procedures, such as endoscopic discectomy, minimally invasive laminectomy, and cervical disc arthroplasty, offer the potential for reduced tissue trauma, faster recovery, and improved outcomes compared to traditional open surgeries. These minimally invasive approaches aim to achieve the same treatment goals as traditional open surgeries while minimizing disruption to surrounding tissues and structures.

In conclusion, surgical interventions for specific conditions in neck pain are important treatment options for individuals with severe or progressive symptoms that have not responded to conservative treatments. These surgical procedures aim to address underlying structural issues, alleviate nerve compression, stabilize the spine, and improve overall function and quality of life. By understanding the specific conditions that may require surgical intervention and the available surgical options, healthcare providers and individuals can work together to develop personalized treatment plans that address the specific needs and goals of each patient, ultimately leading to improved outcomes and enhanced well-being.

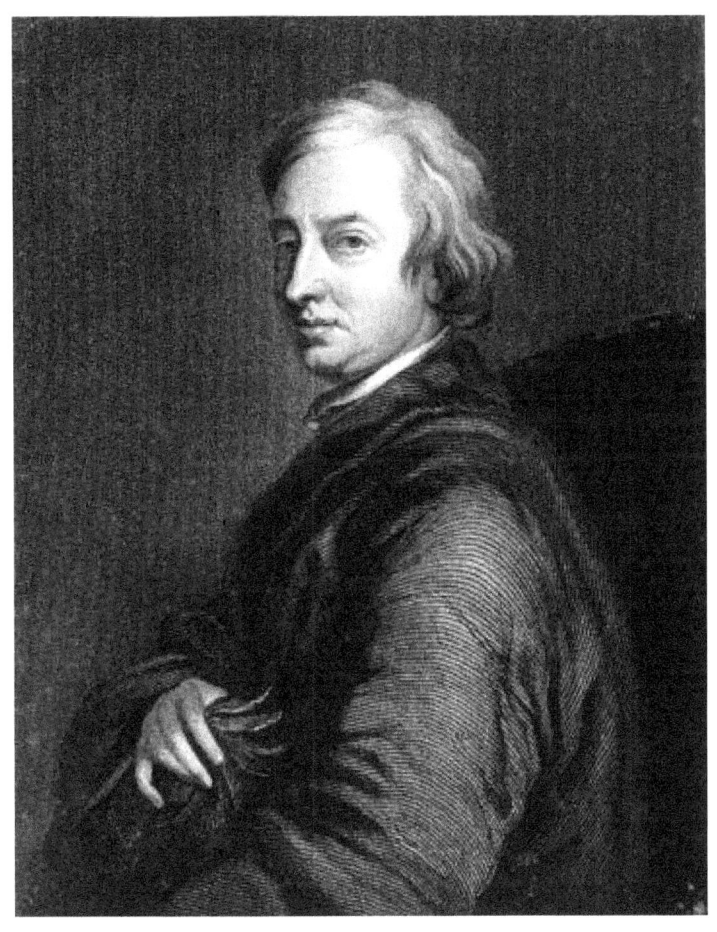

*"For all the happiness mankind can gain: is not in pleasure, but in rest from pain."*
– John Dryden

# Chapter 7

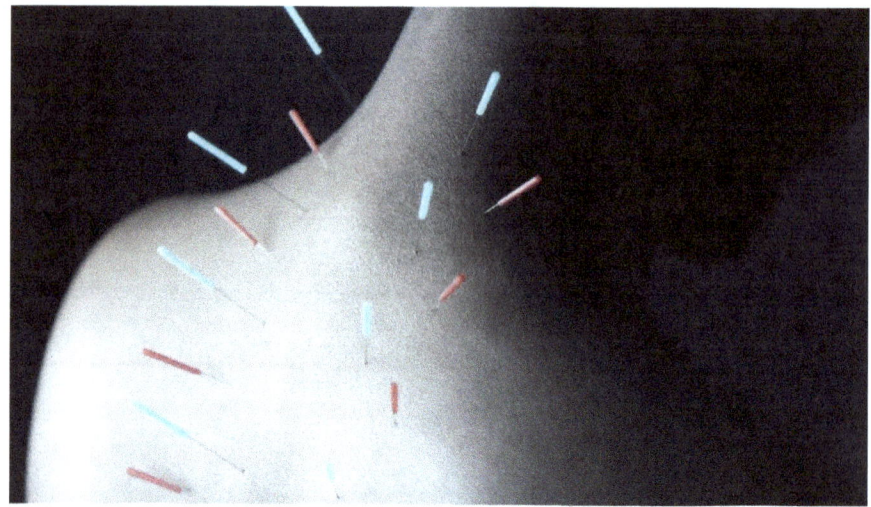

## Complementary and Alternative Therapies

### 1. Acupuncture and acupressure

Acupuncture and acupressure are ancient healing practices that have been used for centuries in traditional Chinese medicine to promote health, alleviate pain, and address a wide range of medical conditions. These complementary and alternative therapies have gained popularity in Western countries as well, and are often sought after for their potential to provide natural and holistic approaches to health and wellness. Understanding the principles, benefits, and considerations of acupuncture and acupressure is essential for both healthcare providers and individuals seeking alternative therapies for various health concerns.

**Acupuncture** is a therapeutic technique that involves the insertion of thin needles into specific points on the body, known as acupoints, to stimulate the flow of energy, or qi, along pathways called meridians. According to traditional Chinese medicine, the balance and flow of qi are essential for maintaining health, and disruptions or imbalances in this energy can lead to pain and illness. By inserting needles at acupoints, acupuncturists aim to restore the proper flow of qi, alleviate pain, and promote overall well-being.

**Acupressure**, on the other hand, is a similar technique that involves applying pressure to acupoints using the fingers, palms, or specialized devices, without the use of needles. This gentle pressure is believed to stimulate the body's natural healing abilities, release muscular tension, and improve the flow of energy throughout the body.

Both acupuncture and acupressure are commonly used to address a variety of health conditions, including chronic pain, musculoskeletal disorders, headaches, stress, anxiety, and nausea. These therapies are often sought after for their potential to provide natural and holistic approaches to health and wellness, and are frequently used as complementary treatments alongside conventional medical care.

Research has shown that acupuncture and acupressure may offer several potential benefits for individuals seeking relief from various health concerns. For example, studies have suggested that acupuncture may help alleviate chronic pain conditions, such as lower back pain, osteoarthritis, and migraines, by stimulating the release of endorphins, the body's natural pain-relieving chemicals, and modulating the perception of pain in the central nervous system. Acupuncture has also been shown to have anti-inflammatory effects, promote relaxation, and improve circulation, which may contribute to its therapeutic benefits for pain and other health conditions.

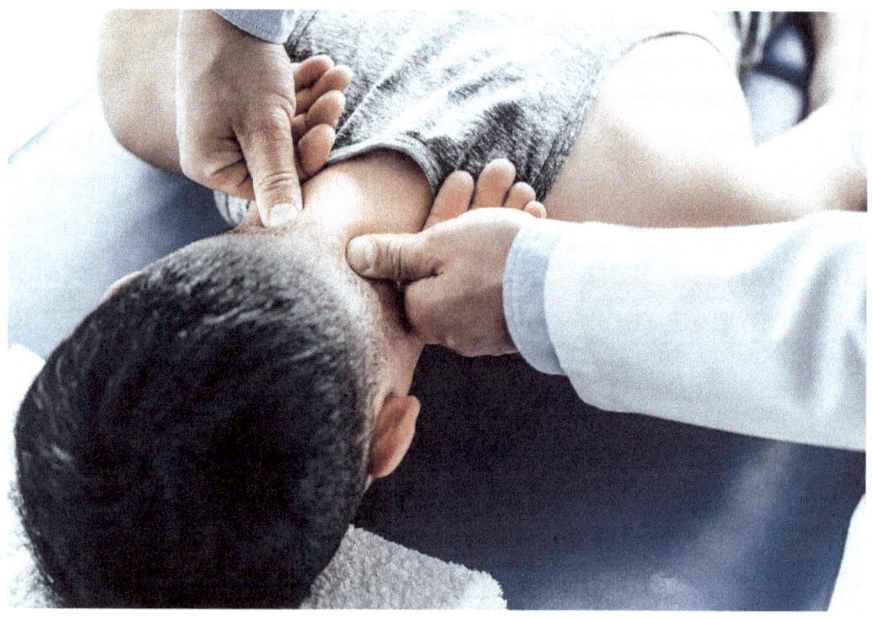

Similarly, acupressure has been found to be effective in reducing pain, muscle tension, and stress, and may offer benefits for individuals with chronic pain conditions, such as fibromyalgia, as well as those experiencing stress-related symptoms, such as anxiety and insomnia. Acupressure techniques, such as Shiatsu and Tui Na, which involve applying rhythmic pressure to acupoints and meridians, have been shown to promote relaxation, improve sleep quality, and enhance overall well-being.

In addition to pain management, acupuncture and acupressure are often used to address nausea and vomiting associated with chemotherapy, pregnancy, and postoperative recovery. Research has indicated that these therapies may help regulate the body's autonomic nervous system, reduce nausea and vomiting, and improve appetite and digestion, offering a natural and complementary approach to managing these common symptoms.

Furthermore, acupuncture and acupressure are frequently used to support mental and emotional well-being, as they are believed to help regulate the body's stress response, promote relaxation, and improve mood. These therapies may be beneficial for individuals experiencing stress, anxiety, depression, and other mood-related concerns, offering a holistic approach to mental health and wellness.

When considering acupuncture and acupressure as complementary and alternative therapies, it is important for individuals to seek qualified practitioners who have received proper training and certification in these techniques. Healthcare providers can help individuals identify reputable acupuncturists and acupressure practitioners who adhere to safety and hygiene standards and follow ethical guidelines in their practice.

In conclusion, acupuncture and acupressure are ancient healing practices that offer potential benefits for individuals seeking natural and holistic approaches to health and wellness. These complementary and alternative therapies have been used for centuries to promote health, alleviate pain, and address a wide range of medical conditions, and are often sought after for their potential to provide natural and effective treatments for various health concerns. By understanding the principles, benefits, and considerations of acupuncture and acupressure, healthcare providers and individuals can explore these therapies as part of a comprehensive approach to health and well-being, ultimately leading to improved outcomes and enhanced quality of life.

## 2. Chiropractic care

Chiropractic care is a popular and widely utilized complementary and alternative therapy for individuals experiencing neck pain. This non-invasive approach to healthcare focuses on the diagnosis, treatment, and prevention of musculoskeletal disorders, with a particular emphasis on the spine. Chiropractors are trained to assess and manage various spinal conditions, including neck pain, through manual adjustments, mobilization techniques, therapeutic exercises, and patient education. Understanding the principles, benefits, and considerations of chiropractic care in the context of neck pain is essential for both healthcare providers and individuals seeking alternative therapies for this common and often debilitating condition.

One of the primary goals of chiropractic care in neck pain management is to address musculoskeletal imbalances, restore proper spinal alignment, and alleviate discomfort. Chiropractors use a hands-on approach to manipulate the spine and surrounding structures, aiming to improve joint function, reduce inflammation, and promote natural healing. By applying controlled force to specific areas of the spine through manual adjustments, chiropractors seek to correct misalignments, or subluxations, that may contribute to neck pain and related symptoms.

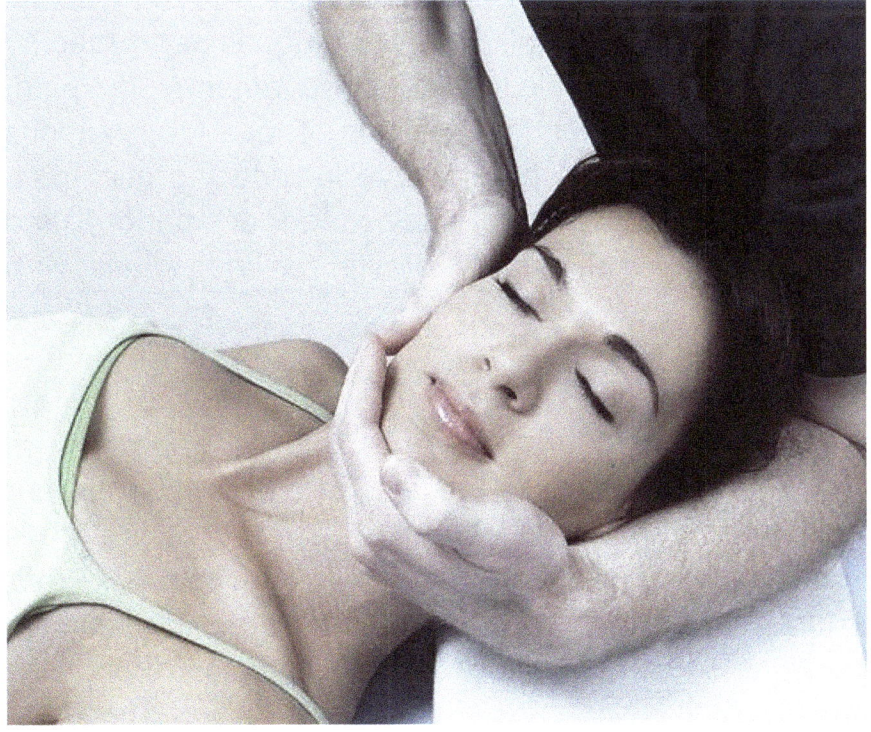

Chiropractic care also emphasizes the importance of spinal mobilization, which involves gentle stretching and movement of the spinal joints to improve range of motion, reduce muscle tension, and enhance flexibility. These techniques aim to restore normal spinal function, alleviate pressure on the nerves, and promote overall musculoskeletal health. Additionally, chiropractors may incorporate therapeutic exercises, such as stretching and strengthening routines, to help individuals improve posture, enhance core stability, and prevent future episodes of neck pain.

Research has shown that chiropractic care may offer several potential benefits for individuals with neck pain. For example, studies have suggested that spinal manipulation and mobilization techniques performed by chiropractors can lead to improvements in pain, function, and patient satisfaction. These interventions have been found to be effective in reducing neck pain intensity, improving cervical range of motion, and enhancing overall quality of life for individuals with acute and chronic neck pain.

Furthermore, chiropractic care is often sought after for its natural and non-pharmacological approach to managing neck pain. By focusing on the body's inherent ability to heal and self-regulate, chiropractors aim to provide conservative and personalized treatments that address the root cause of neck pain, rather than simply masking the symptoms with medication. This holistic approach to healthcare aligns with the preferences of individuals seeking natural and complementary therapies for their health concerns.

In addition to pain management, chiropractic care emphasizes patient education and empowerment, as chiropractors work with individuals to develop strategies for maintaining spinal health and preventing future episodes of neck pain. This may include guidance on proper posture, ergonomics, and lifestyle modifications, as well as recommendations for at-home exercises and self-care techniques to support ongoing musculoskeletal wellness.

When considering chiropractic care as a complementary and alternative therapy for neck pain, it is important for individuals to seek qualified and licensed chiropractors who have received proper training and certification in this field. Healthcare providers can help individuals identify reputable chiropractic practitioners who adhere to safety and ethical standards in their practice.

In conclusion, chiropractic care is a popular and widely utilized complementary and alternative therapy for individuals experiencing neck pain. This non-invasive approach to healthcare focuses on the diagnosis, treatment, and prevention of musculoskeletal disorders, with a particular emphasis on the spine. By understanding the principles, benefits, and considerations of chiropractic care in the context of neck pain, healthcare providers and individuals can explore this holistic approach to musculoskeletal health and well-being, ultimately leading to improved outcomes and enhanced quality of life.

### 3. Mind-body approaches (yoga, meditation)

Mind-body approaches, such as yoga and meditation, have gained recognition as effective complementary therapies for managing neck pain. These holistic practices focus on integrating the mind and body to promote relaxation, reduce stress, improve posture, and enhance overall well-being. Understanding the principles, benefits, and considerations of mind-body approaches in the context of neck pain is essential for both healthcare providers and individuals seeking natural and holistic strategies for alleviating discomfort and promoting optimal musculoskeletal health.

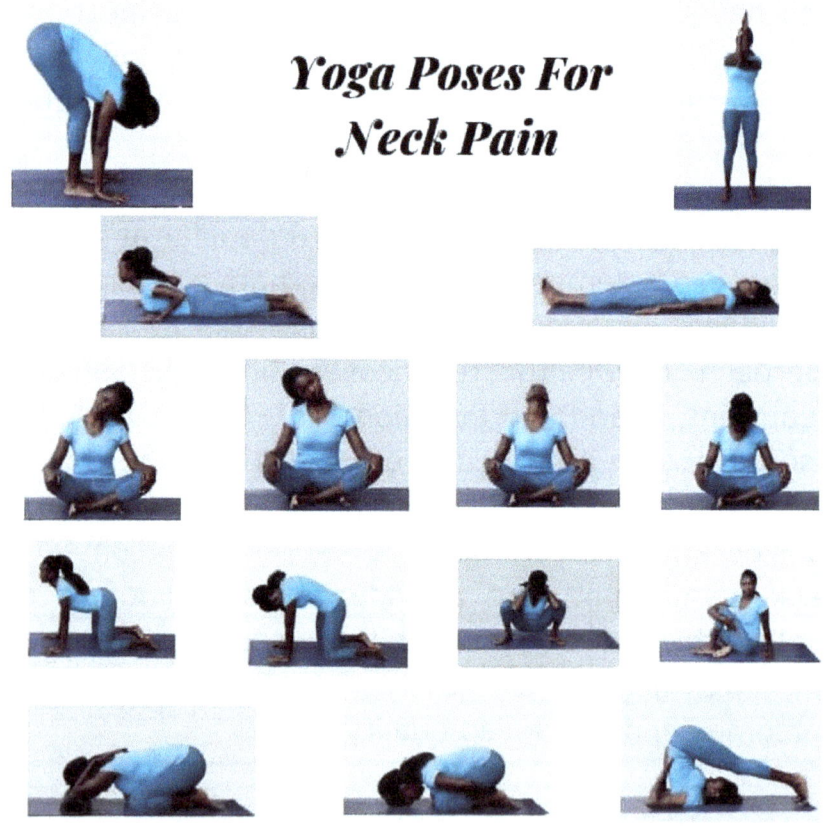

*Yoga Poses For Neck Pain*

Yoga, an ancient practice originating from India, encompasses a variety of physical postures, breathing exercises, and meditation techniques. It is known for its ability to improve flexibility, strength, and balance while fostering a sense of calm and mental clarity. In the context of neck pain, yoga offers specific benefits that can help alleviate discomfort and promote neck health.

One of the primary goals of yoga in neck pain management is to address muscular imbalances, reduce tension, and improve posture. Many yoga poses focus on stretching and strengthening the muscles of the neck, shoulders, and upper back, which can help alleviate muscle tightness and promote proper alignment of the cervical spine. Additionally, yoga emphasizes the importance of breath awareness and relaxation, which can help individuals manage stress and tension, common contributors to neck pain.

Research has shown that yoga may offer several potential benefits for individuals with neck pain. Studies have suggested that regular practice of yoga can lead to improvements in pain, function, and overall quality of life for individuals with acute and chronic neck pain. Yoga has been found to be effective in reducing neck pain intensity, improving cervical range of motion, and enhancing overall well-being.

Meditation, another key component of mind-body approaches, involves training the mind to achieve a state of focused attention and heightened awareness.

It encompasses various techniques, such as mindfulness meditation, guided imagery, and loving-kindness meditation, all of which can be beneficial for individuals with neck pain.

In the context of neck pain, meditation offers a valuable tool for managing stress, reducing muscle tension, and promoting relaxation. By cultivating a sense of mindfulness and present-moment awareness, individuals can learn to observe and release physical and mental tension, which can contribute to the alleviation of neck pain. Additionally, meditation can help individuals develop coping strategies for dealing with the emotional and psychological impact of chronic discomfort.

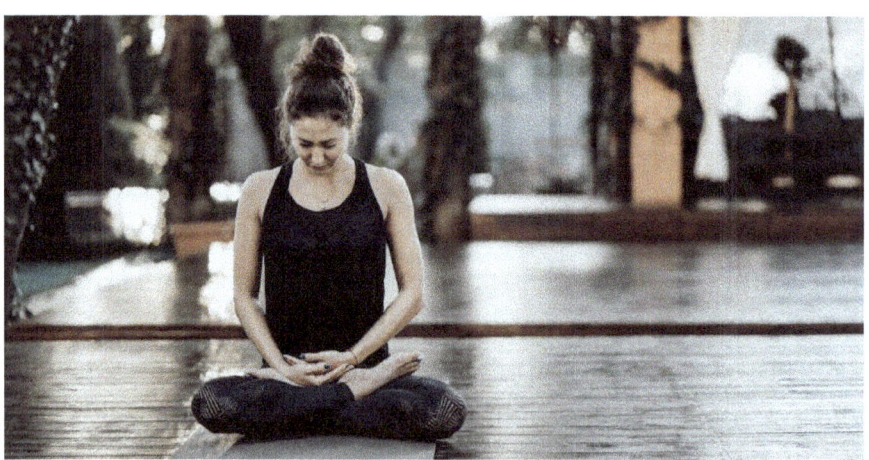

When considering mind-body approaches, such as yoga and meditation, as complementary therapies for neck pain, it is important for individuals to seek qualified instructors or practitioners who have experience working with individuals with musculoskeletal conditions. Healthcare providers can help individuals identify reputable yoga instructors and meditation teachers who can provide guidance and support tailored to their specific needs.

In conclusion, mind-body approaches, such as yoga and meditation, offer valuable strategies for managing neck pain and promoting overall well-being. These holistic practices focus on integrating the mind and body to improve posture, reduce stress, and alleviate discomfort. By understanding the principles, benefits, and considerations of mind-body approaches in the context of neck pain, healthcare providers and individuals can explore these natural and effective strategies to support musculoskeletal health and enhance quality of life.

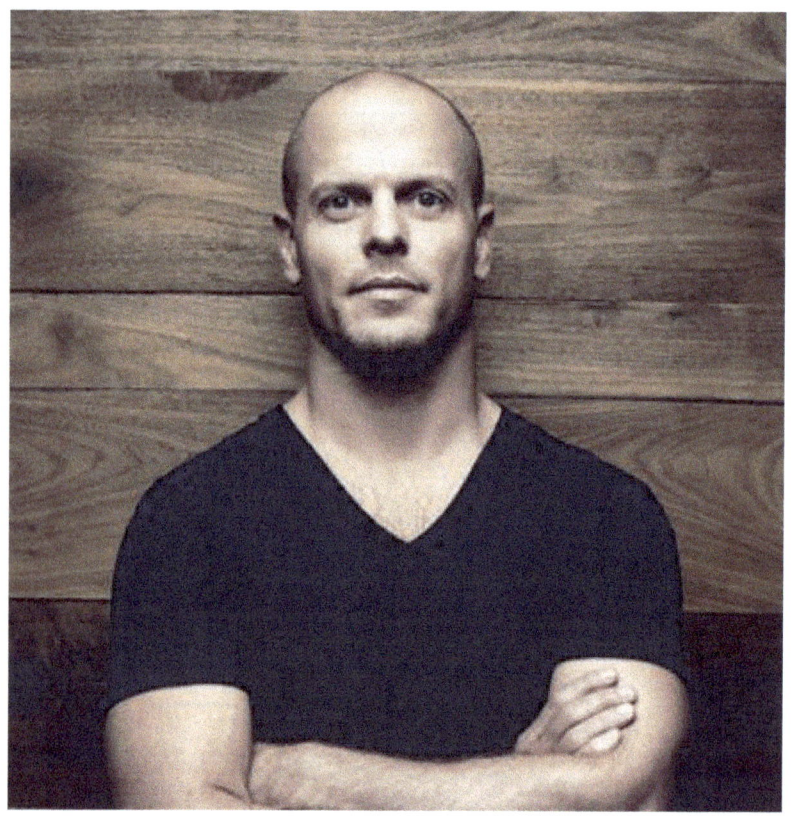

*"When you elevate the heels more so than you elevate the sole of the foot, you trigger a cascade of compensations in the knees and hips that cause tight hip flexors, and then those hip flexors cause back pain."*

- Tim Ferriss

# Chapter 8

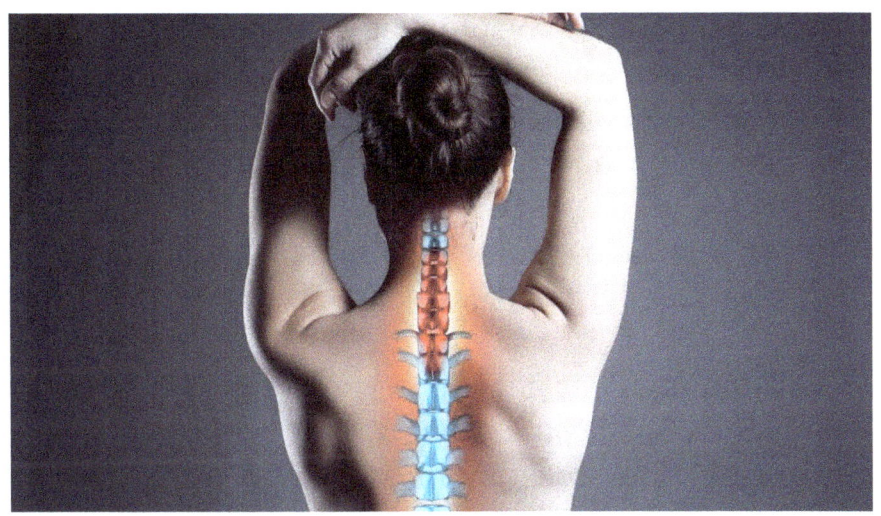

## Psychological and Emotional Impact

### 1. Coping with chronic pain

Coping with chronic pain in the neck can be a challenging and emotionally taxing experience, impacting various aspects of an individual's life. The psychological and emotional impact of chronic neck pain extends beyond physical discomfort, often leading to feelings of frustration, anxiety, depression, and a sense of helplessness. Understanding the complexities of coping with chronic neck pain and addressing its psychological and emotional impact is essential for healthcare providers and individuals seeking effective strategies for managing this pervasive condition.

Chronic neck pain, characterized by persistent discomfort and functional limitations in the neck region, can have profound effects on an individual's mental and emotional well-being. The persistent nature of chronic neck pain can lead to a range of psychological responses, including heightened stress, irritability, and mood disturbances. Individuals may experience a sense of loss, as chronic neck pain can disrupt daily activities, limit mobility, and impact social and occupational functioning. Moreover, the uncertainty of living with ongoing neck pain can contribute to feelings of anxiety, fear, and a diminished sense of control over one's life.

In addition to stress and anxiety, chronic neck pain can also be a significant factor in the development of depression. The constant presence of pain, coupled with its impact on daily life, can lead to feelings of hopelessness, sadness, and a loss of interest in previously enjoyable activities. The emotional toll of chronic neck pain can strain relationships, reduce social engagement, and contribute to a sense of isolation and loneliness.

Coping with chronic neck pain requires a multifaceted approach that addresses both the physical and emotional aspects of the condition. Healthcare providers play a crucial role in supporting individuals with chronic neck pain by acknowledging and addressing the psychological and emotional impact of their condition. By recognizing the interconnected nature of pain and emotional well-being, healthcare providers can offer comprehensive care that encompasses pain management, psychological support, and strategies for enhancing overall quality of life.

One of the key components of coping with chronic neck pain is developing effective pain management strategies that address both the physical and emotional aspects of the condition. This may involve a combination of pharmacological interventions, such as medications for pain relief and mood management, as well as non-pharmacological approaches, including physical therapy, exercise, and complementary therapies. By addressing the physical symptoms of pain, individuals can experience improvements in their overall well-being, which can positively impact their emotional state.

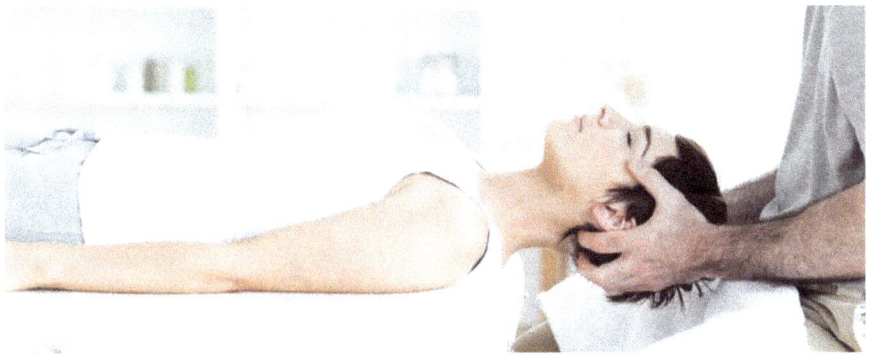

Psychological interventions, such as cognitive-behavioral therapy (CBT), can also play a significant role in helping individuals cope with chronic neck pain. CBT focuses on changing negative thought patterns and behaviors related to pain, promoting adaptive coping strategies, and enhancing problem-solving skills. By addressing maladaptive beliefs about pain and developing effective pain management techniques, individuals can experience improvements in their emotional well-being and overall quality of life.

Furthermore, social support and engagement are essential components of coping with chronic neck pain. Building a strong support network, whether through family, friends, or support groups, can provide individuals with chronic neck pain the opportunity to share their experiences, receive encouragement, and feel less isolated in their journey. Social support can offer emotional validation, practical assistance, and a sense of belonging, all of which are crucial for maintaining resilience in the face of chronic neck pain.

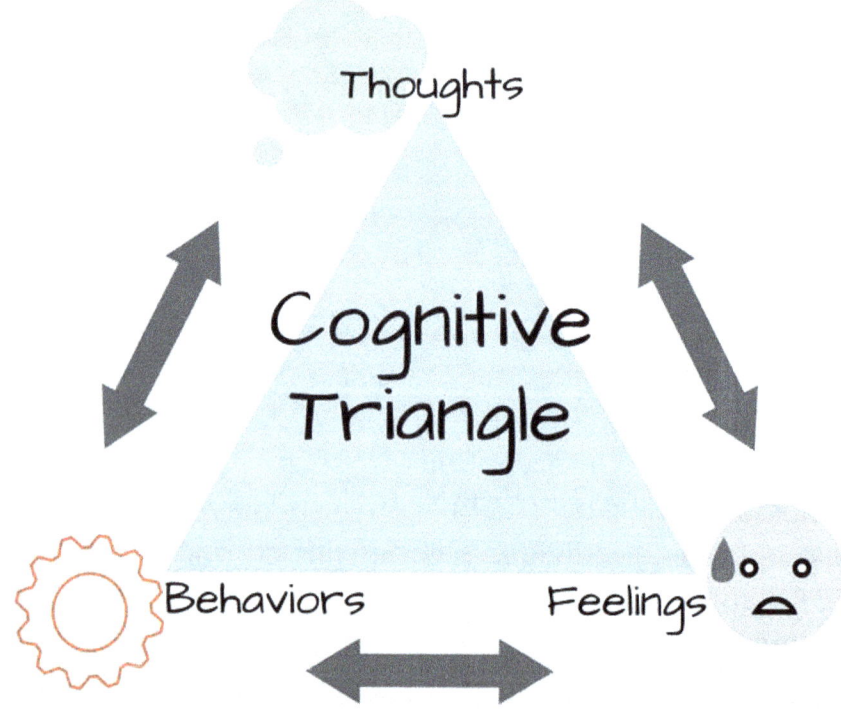

Self-care practices, such as relaxation techniques, mindfulness meditation, and stress management strategies, can also be valuable tools for coping with chronic neck pain. These practices can help individuals reduce stress, manage emotional distress, and promote a sense of calm and well-being. By incorporating self-care into their daily routine, individuals can cultivate resilience and develop effective coping mechanisms for navigating the challenges of chronic neck pain.

In conclusion, coping with chronic neck pain involves addressing its psychological and emotional impact in addition to its physical manifestations. The multifaceted nature of chronic neck pain requires a comprehensive approach that encompasses pain management, psychological support, social engagement, and self-care practices. By recognizing the interconnectedness of pain and emotional well-being, healthcare providers and individuals can work together to develop effective strategies for managing chronic neck pain and enhancing overall quality of life.

## 2. Addressing psychological factors

Addressing psychological factors in neck pain is a crucial aspect of comprehensive care, as the interplay between the mind and body significantly influences an individual's experience of pain and their ability to cope with it. Chronic neck pain, characterized by persistent discomfort and functional limitations in the neck region, can have profound psychological and emotional effects. Understanding and addressing these factors are essential for healthcare providers and individuals seeking effective strategies for managing neck pain and improving overall well-being.

Psychological factors, such as stress, anxiety, depression, and fear, can significantly impact the perception and experience of neck pain. Chronic pain often leads to heightened stress levels, as individuals grapple with the ongoing discomfort and its impact on daily life. The uncertainty of living with persistent neck pain can contribute to feelings of anxiety and fear, especially regarding the potential for exacerbating pain during certain activities. Additionally, the emotional toll of chronic neck pain can lead to mood disturbances, including irritability, sadness, and a diminished interest in previously enjoyable activities. These psychological factors can further exacerbate the experience of pain and contribute to a reduced quality of life.

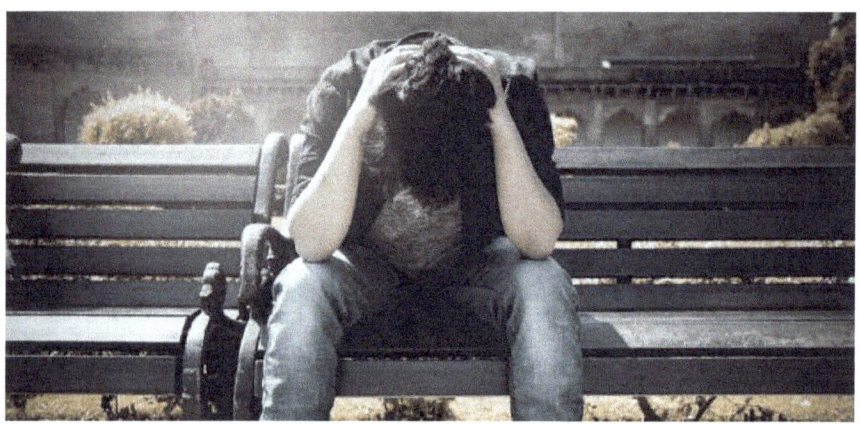

Healthcare providers play a pivotal role in addressing psychological factors in neck pain by adopting a biopsychosocial approach to care. This approach recognizes that pain is influenced by biological, psychological, and social factors, and aims to provide comprehensive, individualized care that addresses the multifaceted nature of neck pain. By acknowledging and addressing the psychological impact of neck pain, healthcare providers can offer tailored interventions that promote emotional well-being and enhance pain management outcomes.

One of the key components of addressing psychological factors in neck pain is the integration of psychological interventions into the treatment plan. Cognitive-behavioral therapy (CBT), for example, is a widely recognized approach that focuses on changing negative thought patterns and behaviors related to pain. In the context of neck pain, CBT can help individuals identify and modify maladaptive beliefs about their condition, develop effective coping strategies, and enhance problem-solving skills. By addressing psychological factors through CBT, individuals can experience improvements in their emotional well-being, pain coping skills, and overall quality of life.

Furthermore, mindfulness-based interventions, such as mindfulness meditation and acceptance and commitment therapy (ACT), can be valuable tools for addressing psychological factors in neck pain. These approaches emphasize present-moment awareness, acceptance of discomfort, and the cultivation of a non-judgmental attitude toward pain. By incorporating mindfulness practices into their daily routine, individuals can learn to manage stress, reduce emotional distress, and develop a more adaptive response to their neck pain. These interventions can help individuals build resilience, improve emotional regulation, and enhance their overall well-being.

In addition to specific psychological interventions, healthcare providers can support individuals with neck pain by promoting self-care practices that address psychological factors. Relaxation techniques, such as deep breathing exercises, progressive muscle relaxation, and guided imagery, can help individuals reduce stress, alleviate muscle tension, and promote a sense of calm. Stress management strategies, including time management, prioritization of tasks, and boundary setting, can also be beneficial in addressing psychological factors that contribute to neck pain. By empowering individuals to incorporate these self-care practices into their daily routine, healthcare providers can help them develop effective coping mechanisms for managing the emotional impact of neck pain.

Social support and engagement are also essential components of addressing psychological factors in neck pain. Building a strong support network, whether through family, friends, or support groups, can provide individuals with chronic neck pain the opportunity to share their experiences, receive encouragement, and feel less isolated in their journey. Social support can offer emotional validation, practical assistance, and a sense of belonging, all of which are crucial for maintaining resilience in the face of chronic neck pain. Healthcare providers can facilitate connections to support resources and encourage individuals to engage in social activities that promote a sense of community and belonging.

Moreover, patient education plays a vital role in addressing psychological factors in neck pain. By providing individuals with a better understanding of the biopsychosocial model of pain, the role of psychological factors in pain perception, and effective coping strategies, healthcare providers can empower them to take an active role in managing their neck pain. Education about the mind-body connection, the impact of stress on pain, and the benefits of psychological interventions can help individuals develop a more comprehensive approach to addressing their neck pain.

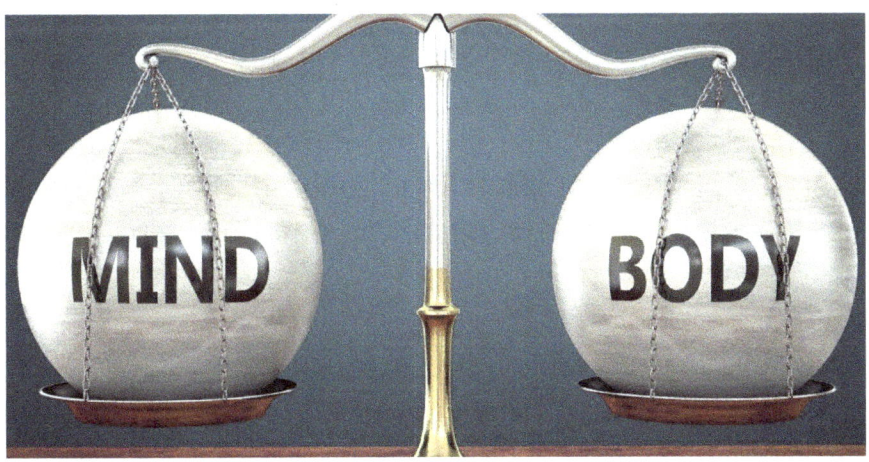

In conclusion, addressing psychological factors in neck pain is essential for providing comprehensive care that promotes emotional well-being and enhances pain management outcomes. By recognizing the impact of stress, anxiety, depression, and fear on the experience of neck pain, healthcare providers can offer tailored interventions that address the psychological and emotional aspects of the condition. Through the integration of psychological interventions, mindfulness-based practices, self-care strategies, social support, and patient education, healthcare providers can support individuals in developing effective coping mechanisms and improving their overall quality of life in the face of chronic neck pain.

## 3. Support for mental well-being

Support for mental well-being in the context of neck pain is a crucial aspect of comprehensive care, as the psychological and emotional impact of chronic discomfort can significantly influence an individual's overall quality of life. Addressing the mental well-being of individuals experiencing neck pain involves recognizing and addressing the multifaceted nature of their experience, providing tailored support, and empowering them to manage the emotional challenges associated with their condition.

Chronic neck pain, characterized by persistent discomfort and functional limitations in the neck region, can have profound effects on an individual's mental and emotional well-being. The persistent nature of neck pain can lead to heightened stress levels as individuals grapple with the ongoing discomfort and its impact on daily life. The uncertainty of living with persistent neck pain can contribute to feelings of anxiety and fear, especially regarding the potential for exacerbating pain during certain activities. Additionally, the emotional toll of chronic neck pain can lead to mood disturbances, including irritability, sadness, and a diminished interest in previously enjoyable activities. These psychological factors can further exacerbate the experience of pain and contribute to a reduced quality of life.

Healthcare providers play a pivotal role in supporting the mental well-being of individuals with neck pain by adopting a biopsychosocial approach to care. This approach recognizes that pain is influenced by biological, psychological, and social factors and aims to provide comprehensive, individualized care that addresses the multifaceted nature of neck pain. By acknowledging and addressing the psychological impact of neck pain, healthcare providers can offer tailored interventions that promote emotional well-being and enhance pain management outcomes.

One of the key components of supporting mental well-being in neck pain is the integration of psychological interventions into the treatment plan. Cognitive-behavioral therapy (CBT), for example, is a widely recognized approach that focuses on changing negative thought patterns and behaviors related to pain. In the context of neck pain, CBT can help individuals identify and modify maladaptive beliefs about their condition, develop effective coping strategies, and enhance problem-solving skills. By addressing psychological factors through CBT, individuals can experience improvements in their emotional well-being, pain coping skills, and overall quality of life.

Furthermore, mindfulness-based interventions, such as mindfulness meditation and acceptance and commitment therapy (ACT), can be valuable tools for supporting mental well-being in neck pain. These approaches emphasize present-moment awareness, acceptance of discomfort, and the cultivation of a non-judgmental attitude toward pain. By incorporating mindfulness practices into their daily routine, individuals can learn to manage stress, reduce emotional distress, and develop a more adaptive response to their neck pain. These interventions can help individuals build resilience, improve emotional regulation, and enhance their overall well-being.

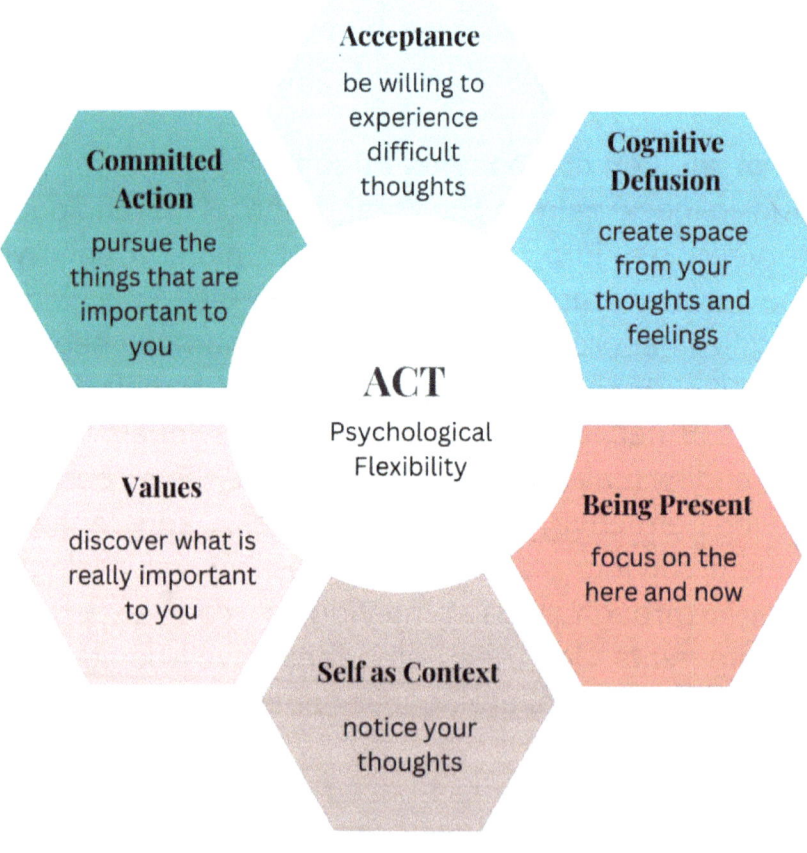

In addition to specific psychological interventions, healthcare providers can support individuals with neck pain by promoting self-care practices that address mental well-being. Relaxation techniques, such as deep breathing exercises, progressive muscle relaxation, and guided imagery, can help individuals reduce stress, alleviate muscle tension, and promote a sense of calm. Stress management strategies, including time management, prioritization of tasks, and boundary setting, can also be beneficial in supporting mental well-being in neck pain. By empowering individuals to incorporate these self-care practices into their daily routine, healthcare providers can help them develop effective coping mechanisms for managing the emotional impact of neck pain.

Social support and engagement are also essential components of supporting mental well-being in neck pain. Building a strong support network, whether through family, friends, or support groups, can provide individuals with chronic neck pain the opportunity to share their experiences, receive encouragement, and feel less isolated in their journey. Social support can offer emotional validation, practical assistance, and a sense of belonging, all of which are crucial for maintaining resilience in the face of chronic neck pain. Healthcare providers can facilitate connections to support resources and encourage individuals to engage in social activities that promote a sense of community and belonging.

Moreover, patient education plays a vital role in supporting mental well-being in neck pain. By providing individuals with a better understanding of the biopsychosocial model of pain, the role of psychological factors in pain perception, and effective coping strategies, healthcare providers can empower them to take an active role in managing their neck pain. Education about the mind-body connection, the impact of stress on pain, and the benefits of psychological interventions can help individuals develop a more comprehensive approach to addressing their neck pain.

In conclusion, supporting mental well-being in neck pain is essential for providing comprehensive care that promotes emotional well-being and enhances pain management outcomes. By recognizing the impact of stress, anxiety, depression, and fear on the experience of neck pain, healthcare providers can offer tailored interventions that address the psychological and emotional aspects of the condition. Through the integration of psychological interventions, mindfulness-based practices, self-care strategies, social support, and patient education, healthcare providers can support individuals in developing effective coping mechanisms and improving their overall quality of life in the face of chronic neck pain.

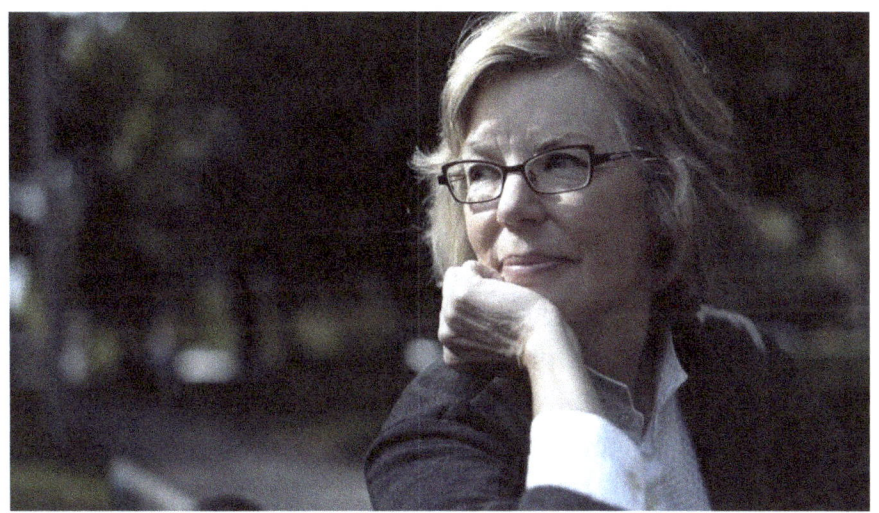

*"Simple intervention – the time spent with a patient – is a very powerful ingredient of the patient-doctor contract. The evidence is against the traditions such as surgery for neck pain being true – the evidence says it doesn't work."*
– Marni Jackson

# Chapter 9

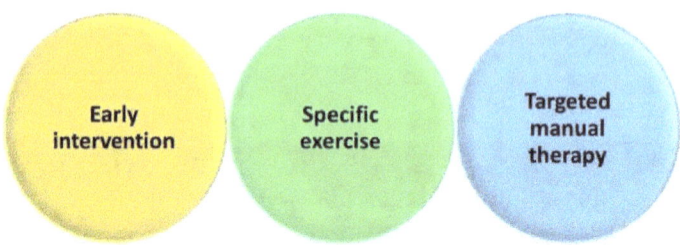

Early intervention

Specific exercise

Targeted manual therapy

## Preventing and Managing Recurrences

### 1. Strategies for preventing future episodes

Preventing and managing recurrences of neck pain is a crucial aspect of comprehensive care, aiming to reduce the frequency and severity of future episodes, improve overall musculoskeletal health, and enhance the quality of life for individuals affected by this common condition. Understanding the principles and benefits of strategies for preventing and managing recurrences in the context of neck pain is essential for both healthcare providers and individuals seeking effective long-term solutions.

One of the key strategies for preventing and managing recurrences of neck pain is to address modifiable risk factors and promote musculoskeletal health through lifestyle modifications. This includes promoting good posture, ergonomic considerations, and regular physical activity. Poor posture and prolonged periods of sitting or standing in awkward positions can contribute to muscle imbalances, strain on the neck and shoulder muscles, and increased risk of recurrent neck pain. Healthcare providers can educate individuals about the importance of maintaining proper posture during daily activities, such as sitting, standing, and lifting, and provide guidance on ergonomic considerations in the workplace and at home. Additionally, incorporating regular physical activity, including neck-specific exercises, stretching routines, and overall strengthening exercises, can help improve muscle strength, flexibility, and endurance, reducing the risk of recurrent neck pain.

Furthermore, promoting weight management and healthy lifestyle habits can contribute to preventing recurrences of neck pain. Excess body weight can place additional strain on the neck and spine, leading to increased stress on the musculoskeletal structures and a higher risk of developing or exacerbating neck pain. Healthcare providers can offer guidance on maintaining a healthy weight through a balanced diet and regular physical activity, which can help reduce the mechanical load on the neck and spine, promoting musculoskeletal health and reducing the risk of recurrent pain.

Another important aspect of preventing and managing recurrences in neck pain is stress management and relaxation techniques. Stress and emotional tension can contribute to muscle tension, exacerbate pain perception, and increase the risk of recurrent neck pain episodes. Healthcare providers can educate individuals about stress management strategies, such as deep breathing exercises, progressive muscle relaxation, mindfulness meditation, and other relaxation techniques, to help reduce emotional distress, alleviate muscle tension, and promote a sense of calm. By incorporating stress management and relaxation practices into their daily routine, individuals can develop effective coping mechanisms for managing stress and reducing the risk of recurrent neck pain.

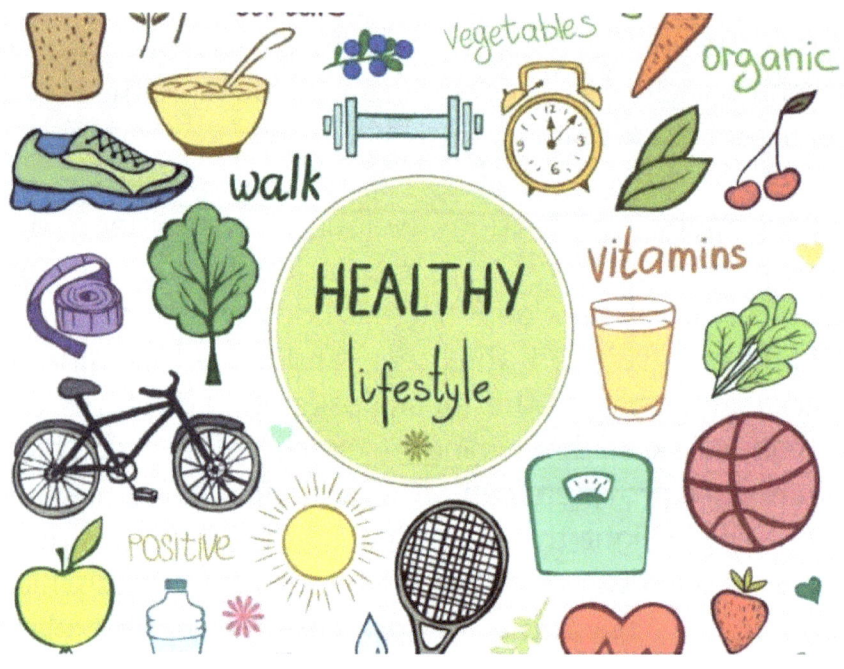

In addition to lifestyle modifications, promoting proper ergonomics in the workplace and at home is essential for preventing recurrences of neck pain. Healthcare providers can offer guidance on optimizing workstations, including proper desk and chair height, computer monitor placement, and keyboard and mouse positioning, to promote neutral postures and reduce strain on the neck and shoulders. Similarly, individuals can be educated about ergonomic considerations in other daily activities, such as lifting, carrying, and performing household tasks, to minimize the risk of developing or exacerbating neck pain.

Moreover, educating individuals about the importance of regular breaks, stretching exercises, and proper body mechanics during activities that involve prolonged sitting, standing, or repetitive movements can help reduce the risk of recurrent neck pain. By incorporating these ergonomic considerations into their daily routines, individuals can minimize the mechanical stress on the neck and spine, promoting musculoskeletal health and reducing the likelihood of experiencing future episodes of pain.

Another important strategy for preventing and managing recurrences in neck pain is to address underlying musculoskeletal imbalances and movement dysfunctions through physical therapy and exercise. Healthcare providers can refer individuals to physical therapists who can assess their musculoskeletal function, identify areas of weakness or imbalance, and develop tailored exercise programs to address these issues. By incorporating targeted exercises to improve posture, strengthen the neck and shoulder muscles, and enhance overall musculoskeletal function, individuals can reduce the risk of recurrent neck pain and improve their long-term musculoskeletal health.

Furthermore, promoting self-care practices, such as regular self-massage, heat or cold therapy, and gentle stretching exercises, can help individuals manage muscle tension, alleviate discomfort, and reduce the risk of recurrent neck pain. Healthcare providers can educate individuals about these self-care techniques and empower them to incorporate these practices into their daily routine to support musculoskeletal health and prevent future episodes of pain.

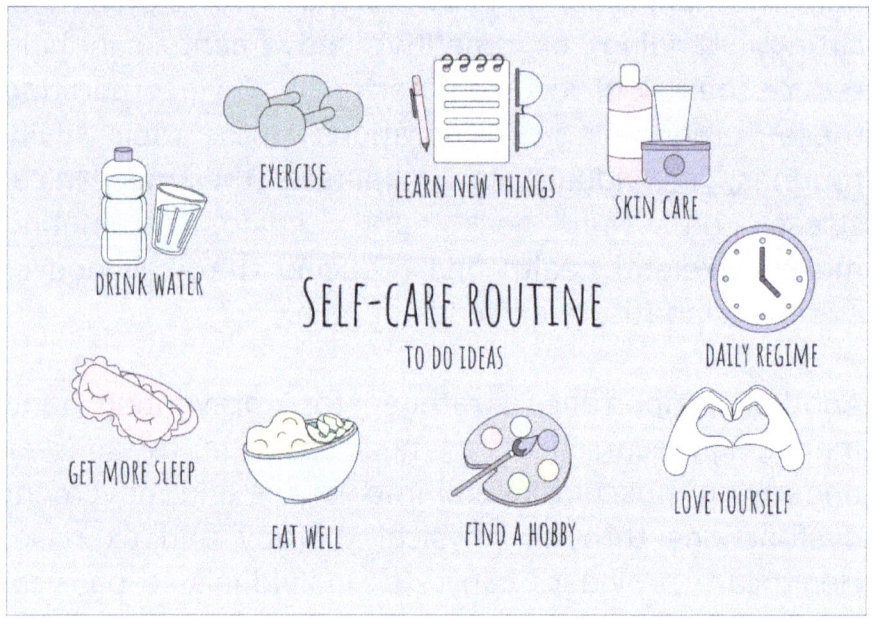

In conclusion, preventing and managing recurrences in neck pain requires a comprehensive approach that addresses modifiable risk factors, promotes musculoskeletal health, and empowers individuals to take an active role in their own well-being. By incorporating lifestyle modifications, stress management techniques, ergonomic considerations, physical therapy and exercise, and self-care practices, individuals can reduce the risk of recurrent neck pain and improve their long-term musculoskeletal health. Healthcare providers play a pivotal role in educating, empowering, and supporting individuals in developing effective strategies for preventing and managing recurrences in neck pain, ultimately enhancing their overall quality of life.

## 2. Rehabilitation and long-term management

Rehabilitation and long-term management play a crucial role in addressing neck pain, aiming to restore function, alleviate discomfort, and enhance overall musculoskeletal health for individuals affected by this common condition. Understanding the principles and benefits of rehabilitation and long-term management in the context of neck pain is essential for both healthcare providers and individuals seeking effective long-term solutions.

Rehabilitation for neck pain encompasses a comprehensive approach that addresses the underlying causes of pain, promotes optimal musculoskeletal function, and empowers individuals to take an active role in their recovery. This may involve a combination of physical therapy, exercise, ergonomic considerations, lifestyle modifications, and self-care practices, tailored to the specific needs and preferences of the individual.

Physical therapy is a cornerstone of rehabilitation for neck pain, as it focuses on restoring mobility, strength, and flexibility in the neck and surrounding musculature. Physical therapists utilize a variety of techniques, including manual therapy, therapeutic exercises, modalities such as heat and cold therapy, and patient education to address musculoskeletal imbalances, improve posture, and promote optimal function in the neck and shoulders. By incorporating targeted exercises to improve posture, strengthen the neck and shoulder muscles, and enhance overall musculoskeletal function, individuals can reduce the risk of recurrent neck pain and improve their long-term musculoskeletal health.

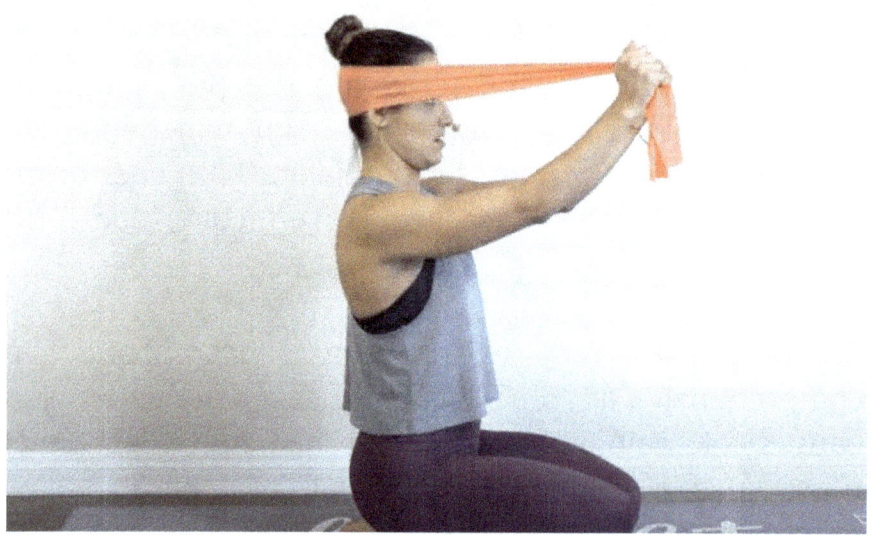

In addition to physical therapy, exercise plays a crucial role in long-term management of neck pain. Regular physical activity, including neck-specific exercises, stretching routines, and overall strengthening exercises, can help improve muscle strength, flexibility, and endurance, reducing the risk of recurrent neck pain. Individuals can work with their healthcare providers and physical therapists to develop a tailored exercise program that addresses their specific needs and goals, promoting musculoskeletal health and reducing the likelihood of experiencing future episodes of pain.

Furthermore, ergonomic considerations are essential in the long-term management of neck pain, as they aim to optimize the physical environment to reduce strain on the neck and upper back. Healthcare providers can offer guidance on maintaining proper posture during daily activities, such as sitting, standing, and lifting, and provide recommendations for optimizing workstations, including proper desk and chair height, computer monitor placement, and keyboard and mouse positioning. By incorporating ergonomic considerations into their daily routines, individuals can minimize the mechanical stress on the neck and spine, promoting musculoskeletal health and reducing the risk of recurrent pain.

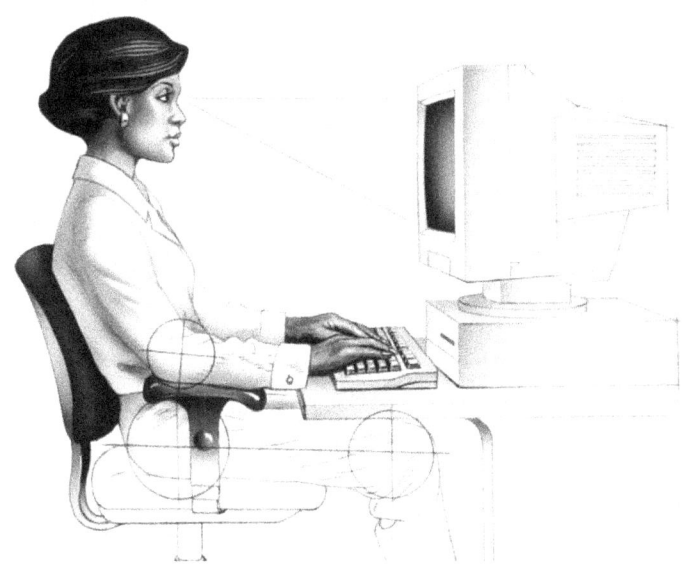

Moreover, promoting self-care practices, such as regular self-massage, heat or cold therapy, and gentle stretching exercises, can help individuals manage muscle tension, alleviate discomfort, and reduce the risk of recurrent neck pain. Healthcare providers can educate individuals about these self-care techniques and empower them to incorporate these practices into their daily routine to support musculoskeletal health and prevent future episodes of pain.

In addition to these interventions, lifestyle modifications are essential for long-term management of neck pain. This includes promoting good posture, regular physical activity, stress management, and healthy lifestyle habits that support optimal musculoskeletal health. Healthcare providers can offer guidance on maintaining a healthy weight through a balanced diet and regular physical activity, which can help reduce the mechanical load on the neck and spine, promoting musculoskeletal health and reducing the risk of recurrent pain.

Furthermore, addressing psychological factors in long-term management of neck pain is crucial. Chronic neck pain can have a significant impact on an individual's mental and emotional well-being, and addressing these aspects is essential for comprehensive care. Healthcare providers can offer support, education, and resources to help individuals cope with the emotional challenges associated with chronic pain, empowering them to develop effective coping mechanisms and improve their overall quality of life.

In conclusion, rehabilitation and long-term management are essential components of comprehensive care for neck pain, aiming to restore function, alleviate discomfort, and enhance overall musculoskeletal health. By incorporating physical therapy, exercise, ergonomic considerations, lifestyle modifications, self-care practices, and addressing psychological factors, individuals can develop effective strategies for long-term management of neck pain, ultimately improving their quality of life and well-being. Healthcare providers play a pivotal role in educating, empowering, and supporting individuals in their journey towards long-term management of neck pain, ultimately enhancing their overall quality of life.

### 3. Red flags and when to seek medical attention
Red flags in the context of neck pain refer to symptoms and signs that may indicate potentially serious underlying conditions requiring prompt medical attention. Understanding these red flags and knowing when to seek medical evaluation is crucial for individuals experiencing neck pain and for healthcare providers assessing and managing patients with this condition. By recognizing red flags and understanding when to seek medical attention, individuals and healthcare providers can ensure timely evaluation, accurate diagnosis, and appropriate management of potentially serious neck pain-related conditions.

One of the primary red flags associated with neck pain is the presence of neurological symptoms, such as weakness, numbness, or tingling in the arms, hands, or fingers. These symptoms may indicate compression or irritation of spinal nerves in the neck, a condition known as cervical radiculopathy. Cervical radiculopathy can result from various causes, including disc herniation, degenerative changes in the spine, or spinal stenosis. When individuals experience persistent or progressive neurological symptoms in conjunction with neck pain, it is essential to seek medical attention promptly to determine the underlying cause and initiate appropriate management.

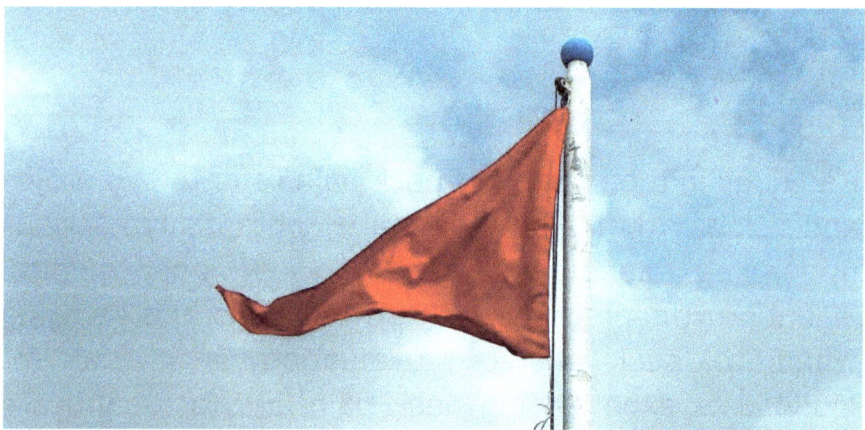

Another red flag in the context of neck pain is the presence of severe or worsening pain that is unresponsive to conservative measures or is accompanied by other concerning symptoms. Severe, unrelenting neck pain that does not improve with rest, over-the-counter pain medications, or other self-care measures may indicate an underlying condition that requires medical evaluation. Additionally, neck pain accompanied by fever, chills, or unexplained weight loss may be indicative of an underlying systemic illness or infection, necessitating timely medical assessment to identify and address the underlying cause.

Furthermore, individuals experiencing neck pain following a traumatic injury, such as a motor vehicle accident, a fall, or a sports-related incident, should seek immediate medical attention, especially if the pain is associated with loss of consciousness, altered mental status, or other concerning symptoms. Traumatic neck injuries can result in various musculoskeletal and neurological complications, including fractures, ligamentous injuries, or spinal cord trauma. Prompt evaluation by a healthcare provider is essential to assess the extent of injury, rule out serious structural damage, and initiate appropriate management to prevent potential long-term complications.

In addition to these red flags, individuals with neck pain accompanied by symptoms such as difficulty walking, loss of bowel or bladder control, or changes in coordination and balance should seek immediate medical attention. These symptoms may indicate potential spinal cord compression or other serious neurological issues that require urgent evaluation and intervention. Similarly, neck pain associated with persistent or severe headaches, especially if accompanied by visual disturbances, dizziness, or nausea, may warrant medical assessment to rule out underlying vascular or neurological conditions.

Moreover, individuals with a history of cancer or immunosuppression who experience new or worsening neck pain should seek medical evaluation, as this may indicate potential metastatic disease, spinal cord compression, or other cancer-related complications. Healthcare providers can conduct a thorough assessment, including imaging studies and laboratory tests, to identify the underlying cause of neck pain in individuals with a history of cancer or compromised immune function, allowing for timely intervention and appropriate management.

## Head and Neck Cancer

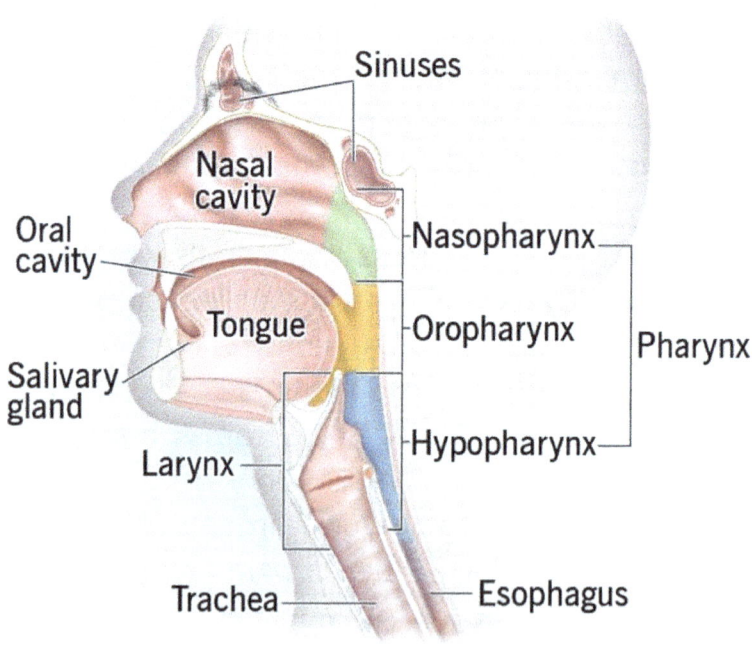

It is important to note that the presence of red flags does not necessarily indicate a serious underlying condition in all cases. However, recognizing these warning signs and seeking timely medical attention can help ensure that potentially serious issues are promptly identified and addressed, leading to better outcomes and reduced risk of long-term complications.

In conclusion, understanding red flags and knowing when to seek medical attention is essential for individuals experiencing neck pain and for healthcare providers involved in the assessment and management of this condition. By recognizing symptoms and signs that may indicate potentially serious underlying conditions, individuals can seek timely evaluation, accurate diagnosis, and appropriate management, ultimately promoting better outcomes and improved quality of life. Healthcare providers play a crucial role in educating patients about red flags, conducting thorough assessments, and facilitating timely intervention when red flags are present, ultimately contributing to the effective management of neck pain and related conditions.

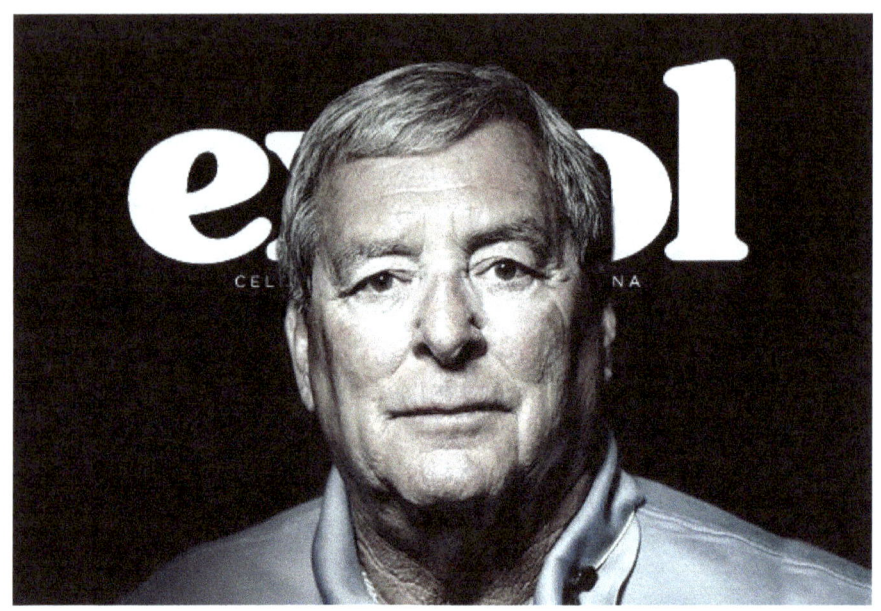

***Vodka does not ease neck pain. But it does get your mind off it.***
— Fuzzy Zoeller

# Chapter 10

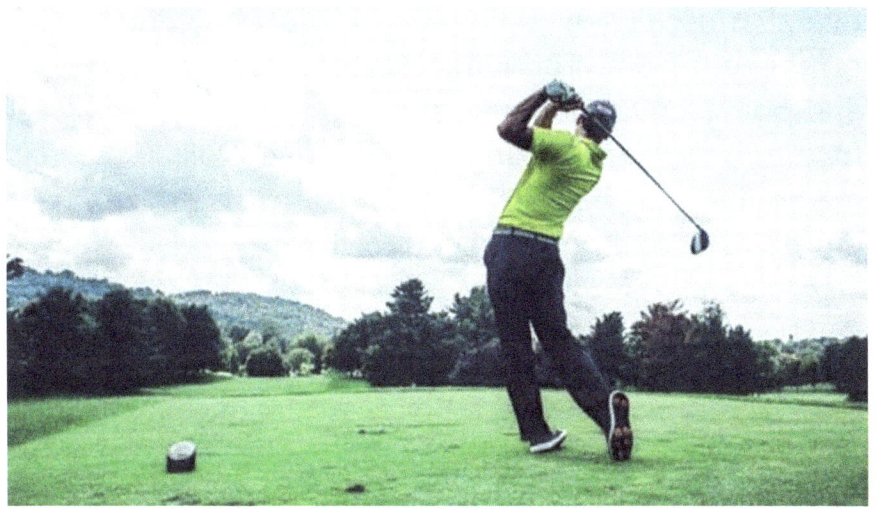

## Living with Neck Pain

### 1. Maintaining quality of life

Living with neck pain can present significant challenges, impacting various aspects of an individual's life. However, by adopting a multifaceted approach that encompasses physical, emotional, and social well-being, individuals can effectively manage their condition and maintain a good quality of life. Understanding the principles and strategies for living with neck pain and maintaining quality of life is essential for individuals affected by this common condition.

One of the key components of maintaining quality of life while living with neck pain is the adoption of self-care practices that promote physical well-being. This may include incorporating gentle neck exercises, stretches, and posture correction techniques into daily routines to improve flexibility, reduce muscle tension, and enhance overall musculoskeletal health. Additionally, individuals can benefit from ergonomic modifications in their work and home environments, such as adjusting computer monitor height, using supportive pillows, and maintaining proper sitting posture, to minimize strain on the neck and upper back.

Furthermore, engaging in regular physical activity, within the limits of one's pain and mobility, can contribute to overall well-being. Low-impact exercises such as walking, swimming, and yoga can help improve circulation, maintain joint mobility, and promote a sense of well-being. It is important for individuals to consult with healthcare providers or physical therapists to develop an exercise regimen that is safe and appropriate for their specific condition.

In addition to physical well-being, addressing the emotional and psychological impact of neck pain is crucial for maintaining quality of life. Chronic pain can take a toll on mental health, leading to feelings of frustration, anxiety, and depression. It is important for individuals to seek emotional support and engage in activities that promote relaxation and stress reduction. Mindfulness practices, meditation, and deep breathing exercises can help individuals manage stress and improve their emotional well-being. Additionally, engaging in enjoyable hobbies, spending time with loved ones, and seeking professional counseling or support groups can provide emotional validation, encouragement, and a sense of connection, all of which are essential for maintaining a good quality of life.

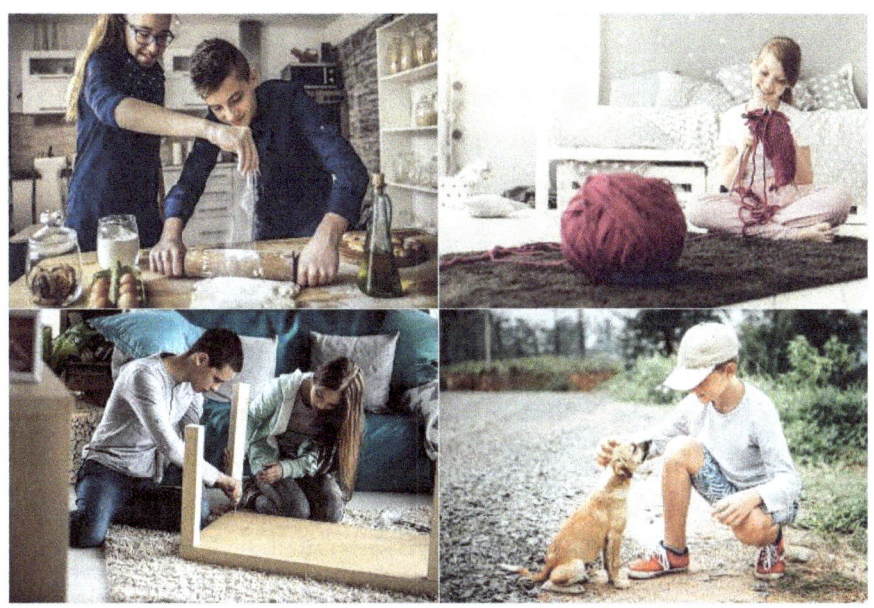

Social support plays a significant role in helping individuals cope with the challenges of living with neck pain. Maintaining open communication with family, friends, and healthcare providers can provide a sense of understanding, empathy, and practical assistance. It is important for individuals to express their needs and limitations to their support network, allowing others to provide meaningful help and encouragement. Furthermore, participating in social activities, community events, and support groups can help individuals feel connected, reduce feelings of isolation, and maintain a sense of normalcy in their lives.

Adopting a positive mindset and cultivating resilience are essential for individuals living with neck pain. While the condition may present challenges, focusing on the aspects of life that bring joy, fulfillment, and purpose can help individuals maintain a good quality of life. Setting realistic goals, celebrating small achievements, and maintaining a sense of hope can contribute to a positive outlook and overall well-being.

In conclusion, living with neck pain and maintaining quality of life requires a comprehensive approach that addresses physical, emotional, and social well-being. By incorporating self-care practices, seeking emotional support, engaging in social activities, and adopting a positive mindset, individuals can effectively manage their condition and enhance their overall quality of life. Healthcare providers play a crucial role in supporting individuals in their journey, providing education, resources, and guidance to help them navigate the challenges of living with neck pain. Ultimately, by embracing a multifaceted approach to well-being, individuals can lead fulfilling lives despite the challenges posed by neck pain.

## 2. Support networks and resources

Support networks and resources play a crucial role in providing assistance, guidance, and encouragement to individuals living with neck pain. These networks encompass a wide range of sources, including healthcare providers, support groups, educational materials, and online communities, all of which contribute to the well-being and empowerment of individuals affected by neck pain. Understanding the significance of support networks and available resources is essential for individuals seeking to effectively manage their condition and improve their quality of life.

Healthcare providers are fundamental members of the support network for individuals with neck pain. They offer medical expertise, personalized treatment plans, and ongoing guidance to help individuals navigate the challenges associated with their condition. Healthcare providers, including primary care physicians, orthopedic specialists, physical therapists, and pain management specialists, play a pivotal role in diagnosing neck pain, providing treatment options, and offering valuable advice on self-care practices, ergonomic modifications, and pain management strategies. By establishing a collaborative relationship with healthcare providers, individuals can receive comprehensive care, tailored to their specific needs, and gain a deeper understanding of their condition and available treatment options.

In addition to healthcare providers, support groups and patient advocacy organizations serve as valuable resources for individuals living with neck pain. Support groups provide a platform for individuals to connect with others who share similar experiences, offering a sense of community, understanding, and emotional support. These groups often facilitate discussions, educational sessions, and social activities, allowing participants to share their stories, exchange coping strategies, and access valuable information about managing neck pain. Patient advocacy organizations also play a critical role in raising awareness, providing educational materials, and advocating for the needs of individuals with neck pain. These organizations offer resources, online forums, and educational events, empowering individuals to become informed advocates for their own health and well-being.

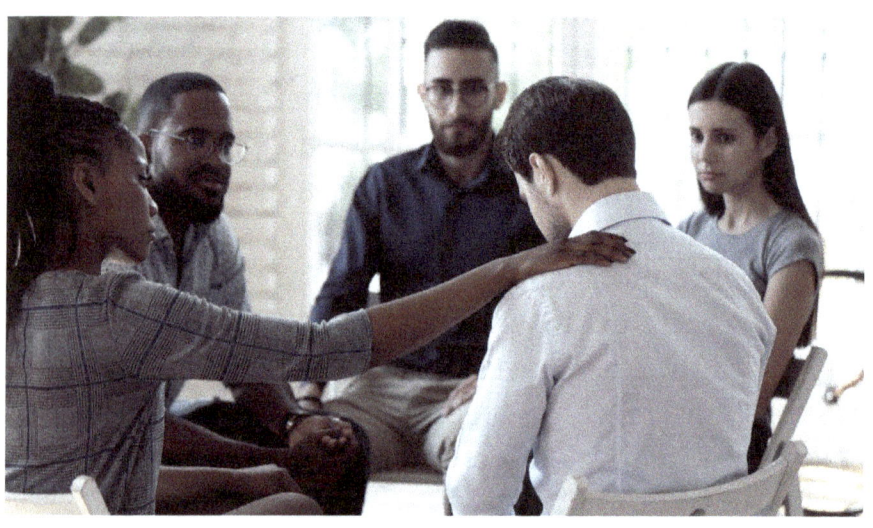

Educational materials and online resources are essential components of the support network for individuals with neck pain. Access to reliable information about the causes, symptoms, treatment options, and self-care strategies for neck pain can empower individuals to make informed decisions about their health. Educational materials, including brochures, pamphlets, and online articles, provide valuable insights into the nature of neck pain, its impact on daily life, and practical tips for managing symptoms. Online resources, such as reputable websites, forums, and social media groups dedicated to neck pain, offer a platform for individuals to access information, connect with others, and engage in discussions about their experiences. These resources can help individuals stay informed, seek advice, and access a supportive community, ultimately enhancing their ability to manage their condition effectively.

Furthermore, mental health professionals and counselors are important resources for individuals living with neck pain, particularly those who experience emotional distress, anxiety, or depression related to their condition. Seeking professional support can provide individuals with coping strategies, emotional validation, and a safe space to address the psychological impact of chronic pain. Mental health professionals can offer counseling, cognitive-behavioral therapy, and mindfulness-based interventions to help individuals develop resilience, improve emotional well-being, and enhance their overall quality of life.

Employers and workplace resources also play a significant role in supporting individuals with neck pain. Employers can provide ergonomic assessments, workplace modifications, and accommodations to help individuals create a more comfortable and supportive work environment. Access to ergonomic furniture, adjustable workstations, and opportunities for breaks and stretching exercises can contribute to reducing strain on the neck and upper back, ultimately promoting better work-related outcomes and overall well-being.

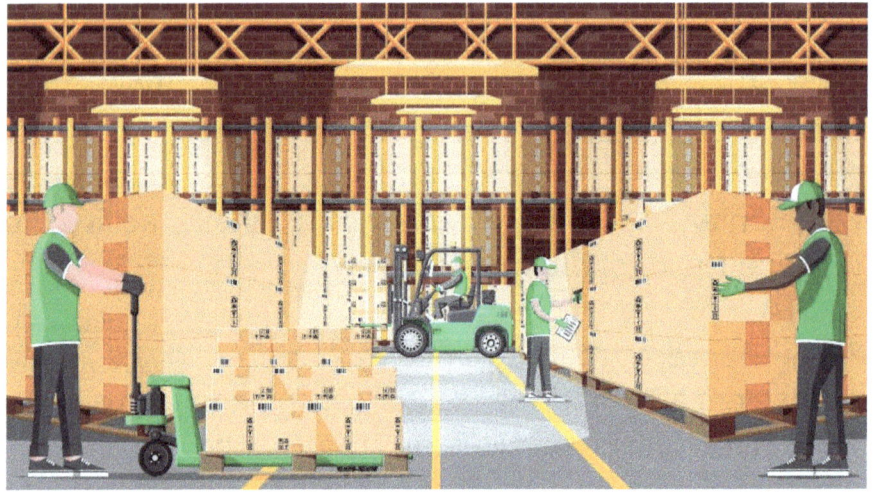

In conclusion, support networks and resources are essential components of the comprehensive care framework for individuals living with neck pain. By leveraging the expertise of healthcare providers, connecting with support groups, accessing educational materials, seeking mental health support, and engaging with workplace resources, individuals can build a strong network of support and empowerment. These resources provide valuable guidance, emotional validation, and practical assistance, ultimately contributing to improved management of neck pain and enhanced quality of life. Healthcare providers, patient advocacy organizations, support groups, educational materials, and workplace resources collectively form a robust support network that empowers individuals to effectively navigate the challenges of living with neck pain and promotes their overall well-being.

## 3. Advocacy and raising awareness

Advocacy and raising awareness play a crucial role in addressing the impact of neck pain on individuals, promoting access to effective care, and fostering understanding and support within communities and healthcare systems. By advocating for the needs of individuals with neck pain and raising awareness about the challenges they face, advocates, healthcare professionals, and organizations can drive positive change, improve resources, and enhance the quality of care for those affected by this condition.

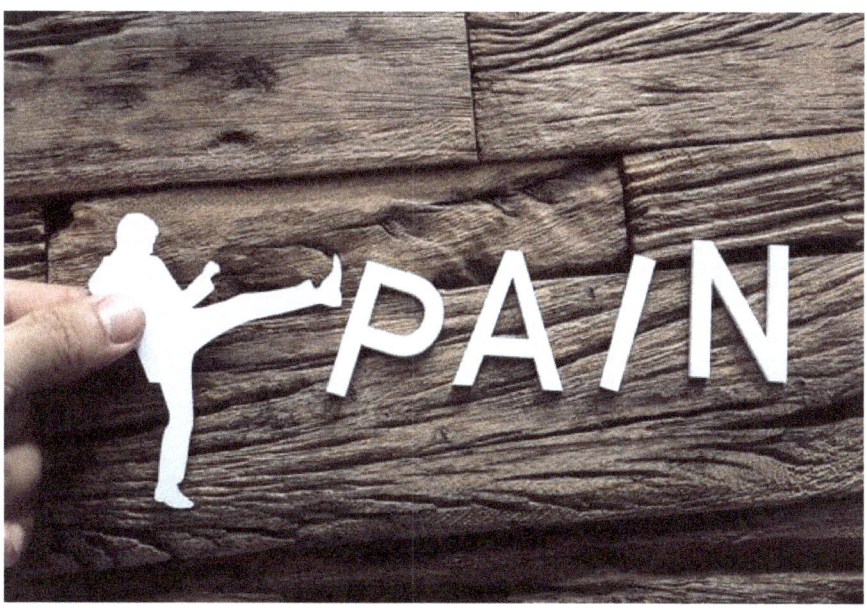

Raising awareness about neck pain is essential for dispelling misconceptions, reducing stigma, and promoting understanding within society. Many individuals may not fully comprehend the impact of neck pain on daily life, including its physical, emotional, and social ramifications. By raising awareness, advocates and organizations can educate the public about the prevalence of neck pain, its potential causes, and the challenges faced by individuals living with this condition. This can help foster empathy, reduce judgment, and encourage supportive attitudes toward those experiencing neck pain.

Advocacy efforts also play a vital role in promoting access to comprehensive care for individuals with neck pain. By advocating for evidence-based treatment options, multidisciplinary care approaches, and improved resources, advocates can help ensure that individuals receive the support and interventions they need to effectively manage their condition. This may involve engaging with policymakers, healthcare institutions, and insurance providers to promote the development of guidelines, programs, and services that address the specific needs of individuals with neck pain.

Furthermore, advocacy efforts can focus on promoting research and innovation in the field of neck pain. By advocating for increased funding for research, clinical trials, and the development of new treatment modalities, advocates can contribute to advancing the understanding of neck pain and expanding the range of available interventions. This can lead to the discovery of novel therapies, improved diagnostic tools, and enhanced strategies for preventing and managing neck pain, ultimately benefiting individuals affected by this condition.

Raising awareness and advocating for the needs of

individuals with neck pain can also contribute to destigmatizing chronic pain conditions and promoting a more inclusive and supportive environment within healthcare settings. By highlighting the impact of neck pain on individuals` lives, advocates can encourage healthcare professionals to adopt a holistic and empathetic approach to care, considering not only the physical aspects of the condition but also its emotional and social implications. This can lead to the development of more patient-centered care models, improved communication between healthcare providers and patients, and the integration of psychosocial support into treatment plans.

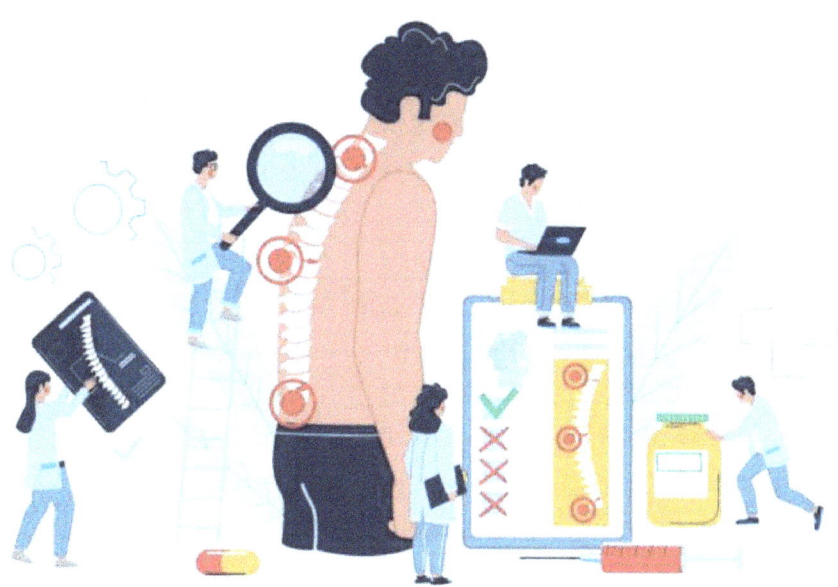

In addition to public awareness campaigns, advocacy efforts can involve collaborating with healthcare organizations, professional societies, and patient advocacy groups to develop educational resources, support programs, and initiatives aimed at empowering individuals with neck pain. These resources may include informational materials, self-management tools, and access to support networks, all of which can help individuals navigate their condition, access reliable information, and connect with others who share similar experiences.

Advocacy and awareness initiatives can also focus on promoting preventive measures and early intervention strategies for neck pain. By educating the public about ergonomic practices, healthy lifestyle habits, and the importance of early assessment and treatment, advocates can empower individuals to take proactive steps to reduce the risk of developing neck pain and seek timely care when symptoms arise. This can contribute to reducing the overall burden of neck pain and improving outcomes for affected individuals.

Moreover, advocacy efforts can address the social and economic impact of neck pain, advocating for policies and workplace practices that support individuals with this condition. This may involve promoting workplace accommodations, disability accommodations, and access to rehabilitation services to help individuals with neck pain maintain employment, participate in daily activities, and lead fulfilling lives.

In conclusion, advocacy and raising awareness are essential components of efforts to address the impact of neck pain, improve care, and support individuals affected by this condition. By advocating for the needs of individuals with neck pain, raising awareness about the challenges they face, promoting access to comprehensive care, and fostering understanding and support within communities and healthcare systems, advocates and organizations can contribute to positive change, improved resources, and enhanced quality of life for those living with neck pain. Through collaborative efforts, advocacy, and awareness initiatives, it is possible to create a more supportive, inclusive, and informed environment for individuals affected by neck pain, ultimately promoting their well-being and improving their overall quality of life.

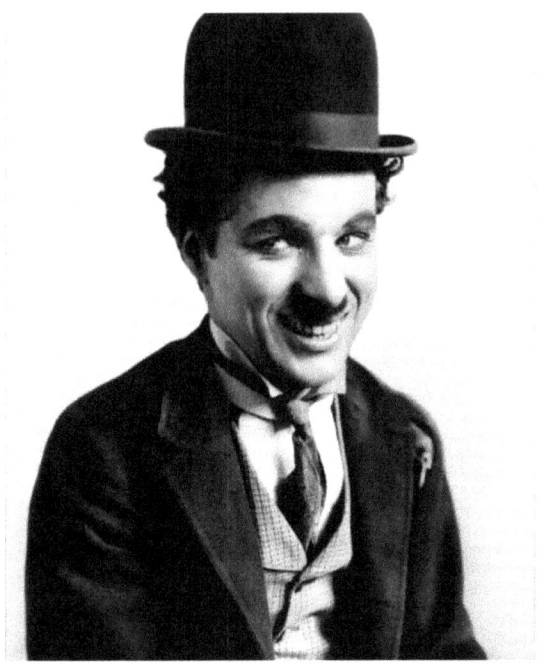

*Laughter is the tonic, the relief, the surcease for pain.*

— Charlie Chaplin

# Epilogue

As we conclude this journey through the intricate landscape of neck pain, it is essential to reflect on the profound impact this condition has on individuals and the broader healthcare community. Neck pain, with its diverse causes and far-reaching consequences, is a complex and multifaceted challenge that demands our continued attention and innovation.

Throughout this book, we have strived to provide a comprehensive understanding of neck pain, from its anatomical underpinnings to its far-reaching effects on physical and emotional well-being. We have explored the myriad factors that can contribute to neck pain, recognizing that each person's experience is unique and may be influenced by a combination of biological, psychological, and social factors. By unraveling the complexities of neck pain, we aim to empower individuals with the knowledge and tools they need to navigate their journey toward relief and recovery.

It is crucial to acknowledge that the management of neck pain is not a one-size-fits-all endeavor. Rather, it requires a personalized and multidisciplinary approach that considers the individual's unique circumstances, preferences, and goals. Healthcare professionals play a pivotal role in guiding patients through this process, offering expertise, support, and compassion along the way. By fostering open and collaborative relationships between patients and their care teams, we can cultivate a more holistic and patient-centered approach to managing neck pain.

Looking ahead, it is clear that there is much work to be done in advancing our understanding and treatment of neck pain. Research efforts aimed at unraveling the underlying mechanisms of neck pain, identifying novel therapeutic targets, and refining existing interventions are crucial for driving progress in this field. Moreover, initiatives focused on promoting public awareness, education, and prevention can help mitigate the burden of neck pain on individuals and society as a whole.

As we strive for progress, it is imperative to remember the human faces behind the statistics and research findings. Each person grappling with neck pain has a unique story, a distinct set of challenges, and a profound desire for relief and restoration. By centering our efforts on the needs and experiences of individuals affected by neck pain, we can foster a more compassionate, empathetic, and effective approach to care.

In closing, I extend my deepest gratitude to the individuals, healthcare professionals, and researchers who have contributed their expertise and insights to this book. Their dedication and commitment to improving the lives of those affected by neck pain have been instrumental in shaping the content and vision of this work.

May this book serve as a beacon of knowledge, empowerment, and hope for individuals navigating the complexities of neck pain, and may it inspire 8continued progress and compassion in the broader pursuit of enhancing the well-being of all.

*Sincerely,*

*Branko Weitzmann*

# Acknowledgments

The completion of this book, „Unraveling Neck Pain: A Comprehensive Guide to Understanding and Overcoming Neck Pain," has been a collaborative effort that would not have been possible without the contributions and support of numerous individuals and organizations. As I reflect on the journey of creating this work, I am deeply grateful for the invaluable assistance and inspiration provided by those who have played a pivotal role in its development.

First and foremost, I extend my heartfelt appreciation to the individuals who have shared their lived experiences with neck pain. Your willingness to open up about the challenges, triumphs, and resilience you have demonstrated in the face of neck pain has been a profound source of motivation and insight. Your stories have illuminated the human side of this condition, reminding us of the profound impact it has on individuals and families. Your courage and generosity in sharing your experiences have been instrumental in shaping the content and spirit of this book.

I am indebted to the healthcare professionals who have dedicated their expertise, time, and passion to the care of individuals with neck pain. Your unwavering commitment to improving the lives of your patients, as well as your willingness to share your clinical insights and research findings, have been invaluable in shaping the content of this book. Your dedication to advancing the field of neck pain management and your compassionate approach to patient care serve as a beacon of inspiration for all.

I would like to express my gratitude to the researchers and scholars whose groundbreaking work has expanded our understanding of the mechanisms, diagnosis, and treatment of neck pain. Your contributions to the scientific literature have provided a solid foundation upon which this book is built. Your commitment to advancing knowledge in the field of neck pain has been instrumental in shaping the evidence-based approach that underpins this work.

I extend my thanks to the publishing team whose expertise and dedication have been instrumental in bringing this book to fruition. Your guidance, support, and commitment to excellence have been invaluable throughout the entire process.

I am deeply grateful to my family and friends for their unwavering support, understanding, and encouragement throughout the journey of creating this book. Your belief in the importance of this work and your steadfast support have been a source of strength and inspiration.

Finally, I extend my appreciation to the readers of this book. It is my sincere hope that the information, insights, and perspectives shared within these pages will serve as a valuable resource in your journey toward understanding and overcoming neck pain.

To all who have contributed to the creation of this book, whether through direct collaboration, support, or inspiration, I offer my deepest gratitude. Your contributions have been instrumental in shaping this work, and I am profoundly thankful for the opportunity to embark on this meaningful endeavor with your support.

*Sincerely,*

*Branko Weitzmann*

# More interesting books by Branko Weitzmann

https://www.lulu.com/de/search?page=1&sortBy=RELEVANCE&q=branko+weitzmann&pageSize=10&adult_audience_rating=00

# Appendices

**More interesting books on neck pain:**

1. "Treat Your Own Neck" by Robin McKenzie

2. "The 7-Minute Back Pain Solution: 7 Simple Exercises to Heal Your Back Without Drugs or Surgery in Just Minutes a Day" by Dr. Gerard Girasole and Cara Hartman

3. "Neck Pain: The 7-Day Neck Pain Cure: The Ultimate Guide to Healing Neck Pain and Preventing Future Pain" by Branko Teodorovic

4. "Healing Your Neck and Back Pain Naturally: The Complete Guide to Preventing and Treating Chronic Neck and Back Pain" by Branko Teodorovic

5. "The Neck Connection: A Chiropractic Approach to Headaches, Neck and Back Pain" by Dr. Paul R. Mahler Jr.

6. "The Neck Pain Handbook: Your Guide in Understanding and Treating Neck Pain" by Grant Cooper MD

7. "Yoga for Neck and Shoulder Pain" by Lisa M. Harvey

8. "The Complete Idiot's Guide to Healing Back Pain" by Deborah Mitchell and Branko Teodorovic

9. "The Mind-Body Prescription: Healing the Body, Healing the Pain" by John E. Sarno

10. "Neck Pain: Why Your Neck Hurts and What You Can Do About It" by Dr. Branko Teodorovic

## Organizations on neck pain:

1. American Academy of Orthopaedic Surgeons (AAOS) - A professional organization of orthopedic surgeons dedicated to advancing the diagnosis and treatment of musculoskeletal conditions, including neck pain.

2. American Physical Therapy Association (APTA) - A national professional organization representing physical therapists, physical therapist assistants, and students. They provide resources and information on physical therapy treatments for neck pain.

3. American Chiropractic Association (ACA) - A professional organization representing chiropractors in the United States. They focus on promoting the highest standards of ethics and patient care in chiropractic practice, including the treatment of neck pain.

4. North American Spine Society (NASS) - An organization dedicated to fostering the highest quality, evidence-based and ethical spine care for patients. They provide resources and education on spine health, including neck pain.

5. American Chronic Pain Association (ACPA) - A nonprofit organization that provides support and education to individuals living with chronic pain, including neck pain, and their families.

6. National Institute of Neurological Disorders and Stroke (NINDS) - A part of the National Institutes of Health (NIH) that conducts and supports research on disorders of the brain and nervous system, including neck pain and related conditions.

7. American Pain Society (APS) - A multidisciplinary professional organization dedicated to advancing pain research and treatment. They provide resources and education on various aspects of pain, including neck pain.

8. American Academy of Pain Medicine (AAPM) - An organization of physicians with a primary focus on the practice of pain medicine. They provide resources and education on the diagnosis and treatment of various pain conditions, including neck pain.

9. <u>American Occupational Therapy Association</u> (AOTA) - A professional organization representing occupational therapists and occupational therapy assistants. They provide resources and information on occupational therapy interventions for individuals with neck pain.

10. <u>World Federation of Chiropractic</u> (WFC) - An international organization representing national chiropractic associations around the world. They promote the highest standards of chiropractic practice and provide resources on spinal health, including neck pain.

**Websites on neck pain:**

1. <u>Mayo Clinic</u> (mayoclinic.org) - A reputable medical website providing comprehensive information on neck pain, including causes, symptoms, diagnosis, and treatment options.

2. <u>WebMD</u> (webmd.com) - A popular health information website offering articles, videos, and tools related to neck pain, covering topics such as exercises, treatments, and prevention.

3. <u>Spine-health</u> (spine-health.com) - An online resource for back and neck pain, offering articles, videos, and forums where individuals can learn about various conditions and treatment options.

4. National Institute of Neurological Disorders and Stroke (NINDS) (ninds.nih.gov) - The NINDS website provides in-depth information on neurological disorders, including neck pain, and offers resources for patients, caregivers, and healthcare professionals.

5. American Academy of Orthopaedic Surgeons (AAOS) (aaos.org) - The official website of the AAOS provides information on neck pain, treatment options, and resources for finding orthopedic surgeons specializing in neck conditions.

6. American Chiropractic Association (ACA) (acatoday.org) - The ACA website offers information on chiropractic care for neck pain, including articles, research, and a directory of chiropractors.

7. American Physical Therapy Association (APTA) (apta.org) - The APTA website provides resources on physical therapy for neck pain, including information on exercises, stretches, and finding a physical therapist.

8. Spine Universe (spineuniverse.com) - An online resource for individuals with spine-related conditions, offering articles, videos, and interactive tools for understanding and managing neck pain.

9. Healthline (healthline.com) - A comprehensive health information website covering various aspects of neck pain, including causes, symptoms, and treatment options, as well as lifestyle and home remedies.

10. Patient.info (patient.info) - A website offering information on various health conditions, including neck pain, with articles written and reviewed by healthcare professionals, as well as a supportive community forum for individuals seeking advice and sharing experiences.

**YouTube Channels on neck pain:**

1. Physical Therapy Video - This channel offers a variety of exercises and stretches specifically targeted at relieving neck pain and improving neck mobility. The videos are often led by experienced physical therapists and provide clear demonstrations and explanations.

2. Bob & Brad - Known as the "Most Famous Physical Therapists on the Internet," Bob and Brad's channel covers a wide range of topics related to physical therapy and pain relief. They have numerous videos dedicated to neck pain, including exercises, self-massage techniques, and posture correction tips.

3. Dr. Jo - Dr. Jo's channel features instructional videos on exercises and stretches for various types of pain, including neck pain. Her videos are informative and easy to follow, and she often provides modifications for different fitness levels.

4. AskDoctorJo - Another great resource for exercises and stretches to alleviate neck pain. Dr. Jo's channel includes videos on neck strengthening exercises, self-massage techniques, and tips for improving posture to prevent neck discomfort.

5. Physical Therapy Central - This channel offers a range of educational videos on neck pain, including discussions on common causes of neck pain, self-care strategies, and exercises for neck pain relief.

# Exercises

## Neck Streching Exercises

The best way to prevent injury is by having strong, flexible muscles and joints that resist strain and injury. The back and neck like movement. Putting the back in a static position for long periods of time, such as sitting at a computer screen for hours, increases the risk of back or neck strain. The best preventive medicine for neck and back strain is movement. Take frequent breaks away from the computer screen to stretch.

Here are some easy stretching exercises for simple neck pain that can relieve simple cases of neck ache. Some can even be used on the job to relieve neck strain.

- Neck Glide
- Neck Extension
- Neck Rotation
- Lateral Extension
- Shoulder Shrugs
- Tilted Forward Flexion
- Deep Stretching
- Resistance Presses
- Towel Pull

## Neck Glide

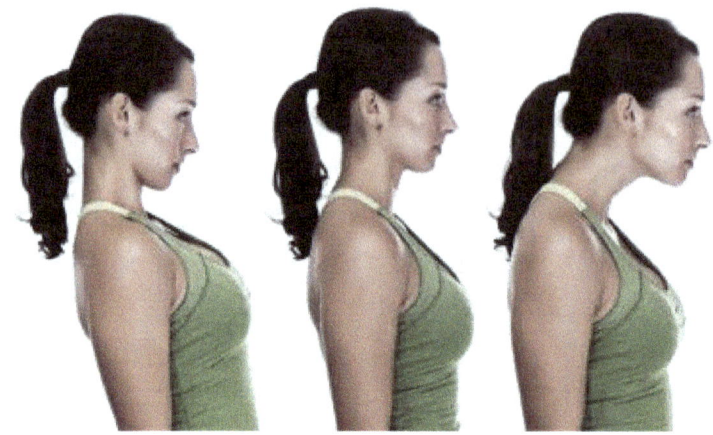

Start with neck straight. Slowly slide your chin forward. Hold for 5 seconds and return to starting position. Do 10 times.

## Neck Extension

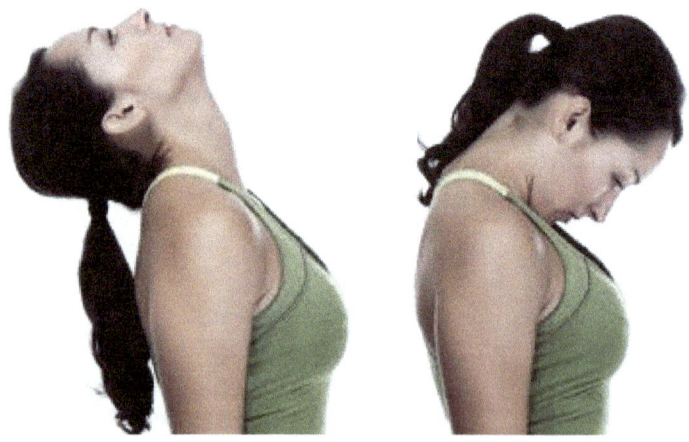

Without arching your back, slowly move your head backward so you are looking upward. Hold for five seconds. Return to starting position. This is a good exercise to do during work to prevent neck strain.

## Neck Rotation

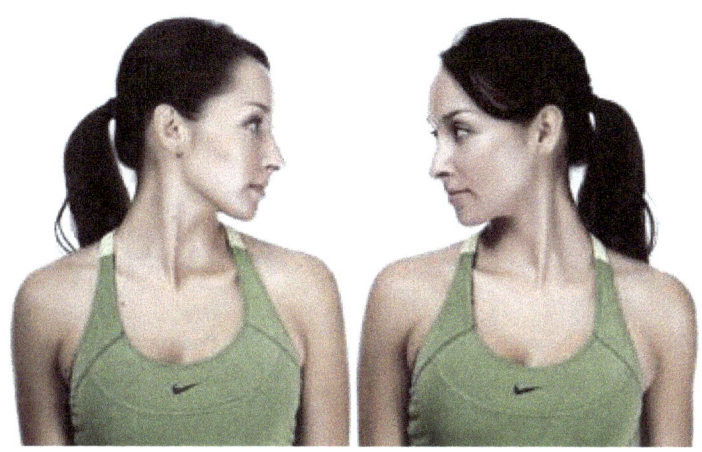

Start by looking straight ahead. Slowly turn your head to the left. Hold for ten seconds, then return to starting position. Then, slowly turn you head to the other side. Hold for 10 seconds. Return to starting position. Do 10 repetitions. This is a good exercise to do during work, especially if you have to keep your head in a steady position for extended periods, as in working at a computer. Do this exercise every half hour to prevent neck strain.

## Lateral Extension

Start by looking straight ahead. Slowly lean your head to the left. Using your left hand for resistance, use the muscles in your neck to press against it. Hold for 5 seconds, then return to starting position. Then, slowly lean your head to the other side. Hold for 5 seconds. Return to starting position. Do ten repetitions. This is a good exercise to do during work, especially if you have to keep your head in a steady position for extended periods, as in working at a computer. Do this exercise every half hour to prevent neck strain.

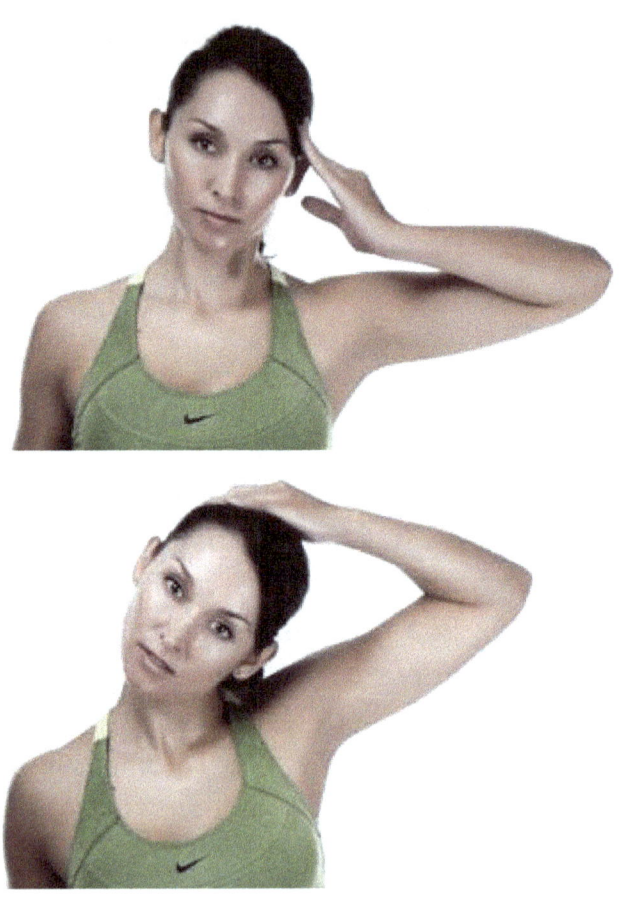

## Shoulder Shrugs

Start by looking straight ahead. Slowly raise both shoulders up. Hold for 5 seconds, then return to starting position. Do 10 repetitions. This is a good exercise to do during work, especially if you have to keep your head in a steady position for extended periods, as in working at a computer. Do this exercise every half hour to prevent neck strain.

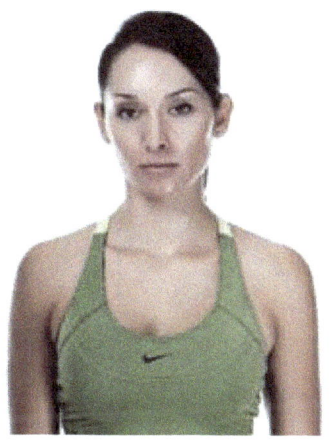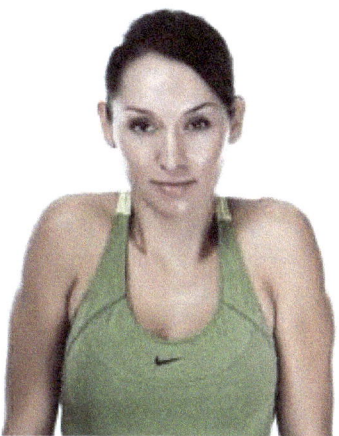

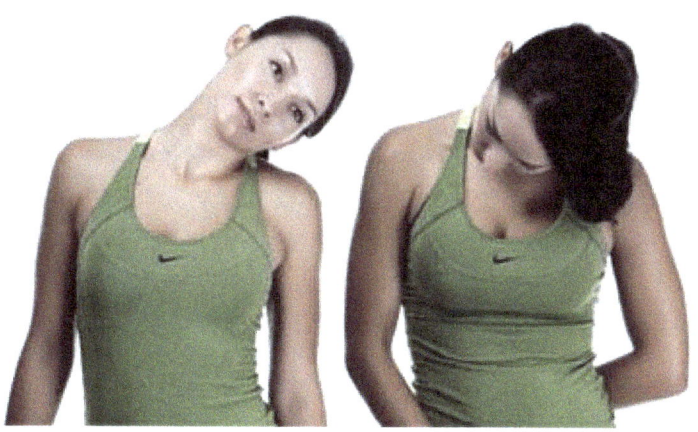

Start by looking straight ahead. Slowly lower your chin toward your chest. Hold for 5 seconds, then return to starting position. Do 10 repetitions. This is a good exercise to do during work, especially if you have to keep your head in a steady position for extended periods, as when working at a computer. Do this exercise every half hour to prevent neck strain.

## Deep Stretching

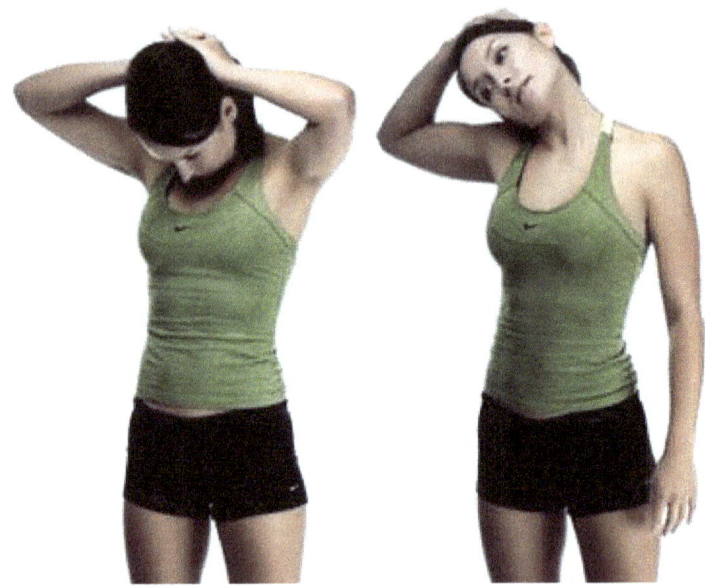

Sitting with good posture, let your head fall towards your shoulder. You can apply pressure with your hand as shown. You may also hold onto your chair with the opposite hand. Hold 30 seconds, repeat 3 times.

## Resistance Presses

Keep your head in a neutral position at all times. Apply pressure to your head in the following positions for 5 seconds then relax. Flexion- place hand at forehead. Extension- place hand at back of head.

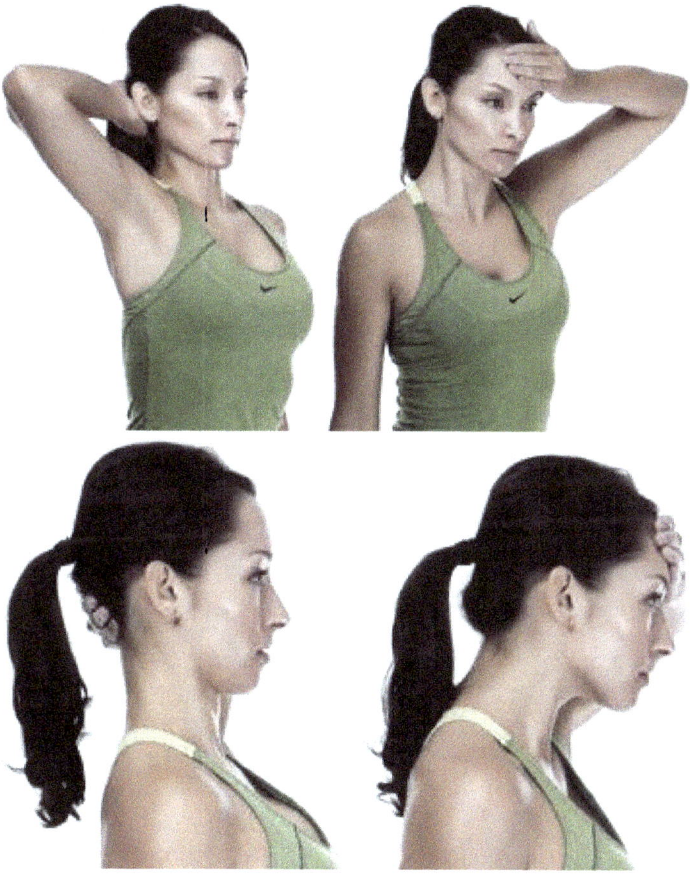

## Towel Pull

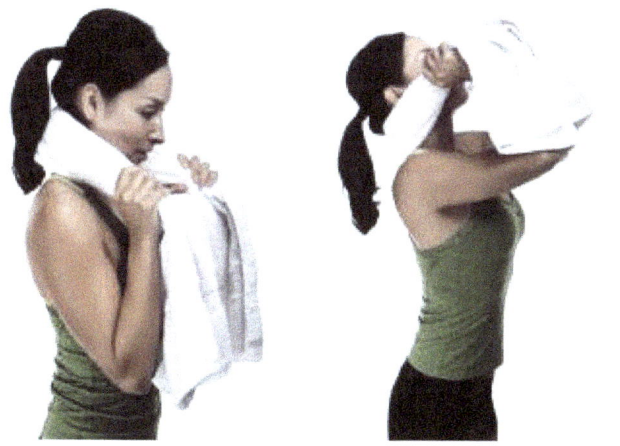

Place rolled towel around your neck, and hold ends with hands. Slowly look up as far as you can, rolling your head over the towel. Apply gentle pressure on towel to support cervical spine as you extend head back. Do not hold the position. Instead, return to starting position. Repeat 10 times.

NOTE: We recognize that people will diagnose and treat themselves. We have provided this medical information to make you more knowledgeable about nonsurgical aspects of care, the role of exercise in your long-term recovery, and injury prevention. In some cases exercise may be inappropriate. Remember, if you diagnose or treat yourself, you assume the responsibility for your actions. You should never do any exercise that causes increased pain. You should never do any exercise that places body weight on a weakened or injured limb or back.

## Strength exercises to relieve neck pain:

Strength training consists of five exercises that involved the use of hand weights to strengthen neck and shoulder muscles. Three times a week (Mondays, Wednesdays, and Fridays), for 20 minutes per session, Do three sets of eight to 12 repetitions (each set lasting 25 to 35 seconds) for each exercise. Increase the weight load gradually, roughly doubling in 10 weeks.

So before you embark on this regimen, consult a physical therapist or exercise specialist who can help design a program for your needs and make sure that you're doing the exercises correctly. In the exercises pictured here, you will find the starting weights in parentheses. For each exercise, you should start with a weight that allows a maximum of eight to 12 repetitions.

## Dumbbell shrug

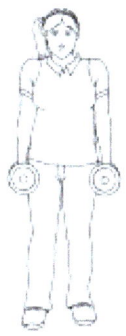

Stand straight with your feet shoulder-width apart and your knees slightly bent. Hold a weight in each hand, and allow your arms to hang down at your sides, with your palms facing your body. Shrug your shoulders upward, contracting the upper trapezius muscle, hold for one count, and lower. Repeat eight to 12 times per set. (Starting weight: 17 to 26 pounds.)

## One-arm row

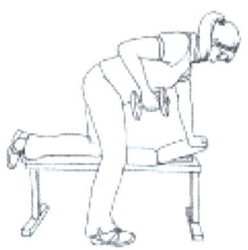

Stand with your left knee on a flat bench and your right foot on the floor. Hold a weight in your right hand. Bend your torso forward, placing your left hand on the bench for support. Allow the weighted hand to hang down toward the floor. Pull the weight up until your upper arm is parallel with your back, pause, and then lower it. Repeat eight to 12 times per set. Switch to the left side, and repeat. (Starting weight: 13 to 22 pounds.)

## Upright row

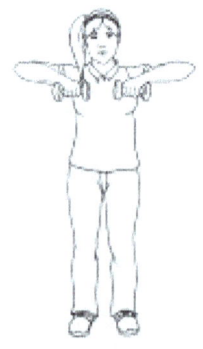

Stand straight with your feet shoulder-width apart. Hold the weights down in front of your thighs, with your palms facing your body. Slowly bring the weights straight up, as if you were zipping up a jacket. Slowly lower the weights to their original position. Repeat eight to 12 times per set. (Starting weight: 4 to 11 pounds.)

## Reverse fly

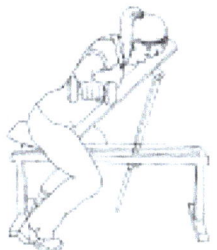

Lie on a bench at a 45-degree angle. Hold a weight in each hand and allow your arms to extend down toward the floor. Keeping your elbows slightly bent, lift the weights up and out to the side to about shoulder level. Slowly lower the weights. Repeat eight to 12 times per set. (Starting weight: 2 to 6 pounds.)

## Lateral raise

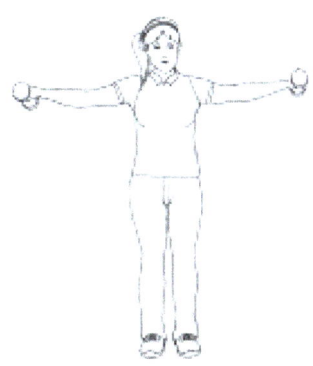

Stand straight with your feet shoulder-width apart and your knees slightly bent. Lift your arms up to the sides until they are parallel with the floor. Your elbows should be slightly bent. Slowly lower your arms. Repeat eight to 12 times per set. (Starting weight: 4 to 9 pounds.)

# References

1. Cohen SP. Epidemiology, diagnosis, and treatment of neck pain. Mayo Clin Proc. 2015;90(2):284–299. [PubMed] [Google Scholar]

2. Ariëns GA, van Mechelen W, Bongers PM, Bouter LM, van der Wal G. Psychosocial risk factors for neck pain: a systematic review. Am J Ind Med. 2001;39(2):180–193. [PubMed] [Google Scholar]

3. Dieleman JL, Cao J, Chapin A, Chen C, Li Z, Liu A, Horst C, Kaldjian A, Matyasz T, Scott KW. US health care spending by payer and health condition, 1996-2016. JAMA. 2020;323(9):863–884. [PMC free article] [PubMed] [Google Scholar]

4. Lezin N, Watkins-Castillo S. The impact of musculoskeletal disorders on Americans-opportunities for action. Burden Musculoskelet Dis US Prev Soc Econ Cost. 2016;3.

5. Safiri S, Kolahi A-A, Hoy D, Buchbinder R, Mansournia MA, Bettampadi D, et al. Global, regional, and national burden of neck pain in the general population, 1990–2017: systematic analysis of the Global Burden of Disease Study 2017. BMJ. 2020;368. [PMC free article] [PubMed]

6. Skelly AC, Chou R, Dettori JR, Turner JA, Friedly JL, Rundell SD, Fu R, Brodt ED, Wasson N, Kantner S, et al. Noninvasive nonpharmacological treatment for chronic pain: a systematic review update. Rockville: Agency for Healthcare Research and Quality (US); 2020. AHRQ Comparative Effectiveness Reviews. [PubMed] [Google Scholar]

7. Li Y, Li S, Jiang J, Yuan S. Effects of yoga on patients with chronic nonspecific neck pain: a PRISMA systematic review and meta-analysis. Medicine (Baltimore). 2019;98(8):–e14649. [PMC free article] [PubMed]

8. Corvillo I, Armijo F, Álvarez-Badillo A, Armijo O, Varela E, Maraver F. Efficacy of aquatic therapy for neck pain: a systematic review. Int J Biometeorol. 2020;64(6):915–925. [PubMed] [Google Scholar]

9. Genebra CVDS, Maciel NM, Bento TPF, Simeão SFAP, Vitta AD. Prevalence and factors associated with neck pain: a population-based study. Braz J Phys Ther. 2017;21(4):274–280. [PMC free article] [PubMed] [Google Scholar]

10. Hogg-Johnson S, van der Velde G, Carroll LJ, Holm LW, Cassidy JD, Guzman J, Côté P, Haldeman S, Ammendolia C, Carragee E, et al. The burden and determinants of neck pain in the general population. Eur Spine J. 2008;17(1):39–51. [PubMed] [Google Scholar]

11. McLean SM, May S, Klaber-Moffett J, Sharp DM, Gardiner E. Risk factors for the onset of non-specific neck pain: a systematic review. J Epidemiol Community Health. 2010;64(7):565–572. [PubMed] [Google Scholar]

12. Kim R, Wiest C, Clark K, Cook C, Horn M. Identifying risk factors for first-episode neck pain: a systematic review. Musculoskelet Sci Pract. 2018;33:77–83. [PubMed] [Google Scholar]

13. Jahre H, Grotle M, Smedbråten K, Dunn KM, Øiestad BE. Risk factors for non-specific neck pain in young adults. A systematic review. BMC Musculoskelet Disord. 2020;21(1):1–12. [PMC free article] [PubMed] [Google Scholar]

14. Linton SJ. A review of psychological risk factors in back and neck pain. Spine. 2000;25(9):1148–1156. [PubMed] [Google Scholar]

15. Martinez-Calderon J, Flores-Cortes M, Morales-Asencio JM, Luque-Suarez A. Which psychological factors are involved in the onset and/or persistence of musculoskeletal pain? An umbrella review of systematic reviews and Meta-analyses of prospective cohort studies. Clin J Pain. 2020;36(8):626–637. [PubMed] [Google Scholar]

16. Xu Y, Wang Y, Chen J, He Y, Zeng Q, Huang Y, et al. The comorbidity of mental and physical disorders with self-reported chronic back or neck pain: results from the China mental health survey. J Affect Disord. 2020;260:334–41. [PubMed]

17. Xie Y, Jun D, Thomas L, Coombes B, Johnston V. Comparing central pain processing in individuals with non-traumatic neck pain and healthy individuals: a systematic review and meta-analysis. J Pain. 2020;21(11-12):1101–24. [PubMed]

18. Ortego G, Villafañe JH, Doménech-García V, Berjano P, Bertozzi L, Herrero P. Is there a relationship between psychological stress or anxiety and chronic nonspecific neck-arm pain in adults? A systematic review and meta-analysis. J Psychosom Res. 2016;90:70–81. [PubMed] [Google Scholar]

19. Mork R, Falkenberg HK, Fostervold KI, Thorud H-MS. Discomfort glare and psychological stress during computer work: subjective responses and associations between neck pain and trapezius muscle blood flow. Int Arch Occup Environ Health. 2020;93(1):29–42. [PubMed] [Google Scholar]

20. Baur H, Grebner S, Blasimann A, Hirschmüller A, Kubosch EJ, Elfering A. Work–family conflict and neck and back pain in surgical nurses. Int J Occup Saf Ergon. 2018;24(1):35–40. [PubMed] [Google Scholar]

21. Liu F, Fang T, Zhou F, Zhao M, Chen M, You J, et al. Association of depression/anxiety symptoms with neck pain: a systematic review and meta-analysis of literature in China. Pain Res Manag. 2018;2018:3259431. [PMC free article] [PubMed]

22. Grimby-Ekman A, Andersson EM, Hagberg M. Analyzing musculoskeletal neck pain, measured as present pain and periods of pain, with three different regression models: a cohort study. BMC Musculoskelet Disord. 2009;10(1):73. [PMC free article] [PubMed] [Google Scholar]

23. Andias R, Silva AG. Psychosocial variables and sleep associated with neck pain in adolescents: a systematic review. Phys Occup Ther Pediatr. 2020;40(2):168–191. [PubMed] [Google Scholar]

24. Jennings EM, Okine BN, Roche M, Finn DP. Stress-induced hyperalgesia. Prog Neurobiol. 2014;121:1–18. [PubMed] [Google Scholar]

25. Lee H, Hübscher M, Moseley GL, Kamper SJ, Traeger AC, Mansell G, McAuley JH. How does pain lead to disability? A systematic review and meta-analysis of mediation studies in people with back and neck pain. Pain. 2015;156(6):988–997. [PubMed] [Google Scholar]

26. Hall AM, Kamper SJ, Maher CG, Latimer J, Ferreira ML, Nicholas MK. Symptoms of depression and stress mediate the effect of pain on disability. Pain. 2011;152(5):1044–1051. [PubMed] [Google Scholar]

27. Ahmed SA, Shantharam G, Eltorai AE, Hartnett DA, Goodman A, Daniels AH. The effect of psychosocial measures of resilience and self-efficacy in patients with neck and lower back pain. Spine J. 2019;19(2):232–237. [PubMed] [Google Scholar]

28. Gureje O. Comorbidity of pain and anxiety disorders. Curr Psychiatry Rep. 2008;10(4):318–322. [PubMed] [Google Scholar]

29. Bobos P, MacDermid J, Nazari G, Furtado R. Psychometric properties of the global rating of change scales in patients with neck disorders: a systematic review with meta-analysis and meta-regression. BMJ Open. 2019;9(11):e033909. [PMC free article] [PubMed]

30. Demyttenaere K, Bruffaerts R, Lee S, Posada-Villa J, Kovess V, Angermeyer MC, Levinson D, de Girolamo G, Nakane H, Mneimneh Z. Mental disorders among persons with chronic back or neck pain: results from the world mental health surveys. Pain. 2007;129(3):332–342. [PubMed] [Google Scholar]

31. Sá S, Silva AG. Repositioning error, pressure pain threshold, catastrophizing and anxiety in adolescents with chronic idiopathic neck pain. Musculoskelet Sci Pract. 2017;30:18–24. [PubMed] [Google Scholar]

32. Kayhan F, Albayrak Gezer İ, Kayhan A, Kitiş S, Gölen M. Mood and anxiety disorders in patients with chronic low back and neck pain caused by disc herniation. Int J Psychiatry Clin Pract. 2016;20(1):19–23. [PubMed] [Google Scholar]

33. Juan W, Rui L, Wei-Wen Z. Chronic neck pain and depression: the mediating role of sleep quality and exercise. Psychol Health Med. 2020;25(8):1029–35. [PubMed]

34. Prins Y, Crous L, Louw Q. A systematic review of posture and psychosocial factors as contributors to upper quadrant musculoskeletal pain in children and adolescents. Physiother Theory Pract. 2008;24(4):221–242. [PubMed] [Google Scholar]

35. Garrigós-Pedrón M, La Touche R, Navarro-Desentre P, Gracia-Naya M, Segura-Ortí E. Widespread mechanical pain hypersensitivity in patients with chronic migraine and temporomandibular disorders: relationship and correlation between psychological and sensorimotor variables. Acta Odontol Scand. 2019;77(3):224–231. [PubMed] [Google Scholar]

36. Mason KJ, O'Neill TW, Lunt M, Jones AK, McBeth J. Psychosocial factors partially mediate the relationship between mechanical hyperalgesia and self-reported pain. Scand J Pain. 2018;18(1):59–69. [PubMed] [Google Scholar]

37. Peterson G, Pihlström N. Factors associated with neck and shoulder pain: a cross-sectional study among 16,000 adults in five county councils in Sweden. BMC Musculoskelet Disord. 2021;22(1):872. [PMC free article] [PubMed] [Google Scholar]

38. Nijs J, Loggia ML, Polli A, Moens M, Huysmans E, Goudman L, Meeus M, Vanderweeën L, Ickmans K, Clauw D. Sleep disturbances and severe stress as glial activators: key targets for treating central sensitization in chronic pain patients? Expert Opin Ther Targets. 2017;21(8):817–826. [PubMed] [Google Scholar]

39. Andreucci M, Campbell P, Dunn KM. Are sleep problems a risk factor for the onset of musculoskeletal pain in children and adolescents? A systematic review. Sleep. 2017;40(7):1–11. [PubMed]

40. Auvinen JP, Tammelin TH, Taimela SP, Zitting PJ, Järvelin M-R, Taanila AM, Karppinen JI. Is insufficient quantity and quality of sleep a risk factor for neck, shoulder and low back pain? A longitudinal study among adolescents. Eur Spine J. 2010;19(4):641–649. [PMC free article] [PubMed] [Google Scholar]

41. Ståhl M, Kautiainen H, El-Metwally A, Häkkinen A, Ylinen J, Salminen JJ, Mikkelsson M. Non-specific neck pain in schoolchildren: prognosis and risk factors for occurrence and persistence. A 4-year follow-up study. PAIN® 2008;137(2):316–322. [PubMed] [Google Scholar]

42. Buitenhuis J, Spanjer J, Fidler V. Recovery from acute whiplash: the role of coping styles. Spine. 2003;28(9):896–901. [PubMed] [Google Scholar]

43. Esteve R, Ramírez-Maestre C, López-Martínez AE. Adjustment to chronic pain: the role of pain acceptance, coping strategies, and pain-related cognitions. Ann Behav Med. 2007;33(2):179–188. [PubMed] [Google Scholar]

44. Wachholtz AB, Pearce MJ, Koenig H. Exploring the relationship between spirituality, coping, and pain. J Behav Med. 2007;30(4):311–318. [PubMed] [Google Scholar]

45. Murugan S, Saravanan P, Avaiya D, Bawa I, Shah C, Vaghasiya E. Prevalence and Risk Factors for Musculoskeletal Pain and Coping Strategies in School Teachers. J Ecophysiol Occup Health. 2021;2021:6. [Google Scholar]

46. Ariëns GA, Bongers PM, Hoogendoorn WE, Houtman IL, van der Wal G, van Mechelen W. High quantitative job demands and low coworker support as risk factors for neck pain: results of a prospective cohort study. Spine. 2001;26(17):1896–1901. [PubMed] [Google Scholar]

47. Haldeman S, Carroll L, Cassidy JD. Findings from the bone and joint decade 2000 to 2010 task force on neck pain and its associated disorders. J Occup Environ Med. 2010;52(4):424–427. [PubMed] [Google Scholar]

48. Moradi-Lakeh M, Forouzanfar MH, Vollset SE, El Bcheraoui C, Daoud F, Afshin A, Charara R, Khalil I, Higashi H, Abd El Razek MM. Burden of musculoskeletal disorders in the eastern Mediterranean region, 1990–2013: findings from the global burden of disease study 2013. Ann Rheum Dis. 2017;76(8):1365–1373. [PMC free article] [PubMed] [Google Scholar]

49. Kuo DT, Tadi P. Cervical Spondylosis. [Updated 2021 Sep 29]. In: StatPearls [Internet]. Treasure Island (FL): StatPearls Publishing; 2021. Available from: https://www.ncbi.nlm.nih.gov/books/NBK551557/.

50. Jiang S-D, Jiang L-S, Dai L-Y. Degenerative cervical spondylolisthesis: a systematic review. Int Orthop. 2011;35(6):869–875. [PMC free article] [PubMed] [Google Scholar]

51. Lebl DR, Bono CM. Update on the diagnosis and management of cervical spondylotic myelopathy. J Am Acad Orthop Surg. 2015;23(11):648–60. [PubMed]

52. Björkegren K, Wallander M-A, Johansson S, Svärdsudd K. General symptom reporting in female fibromyalgia patients and referents: a population-based case-referent study. BMC Public Health. 2009;9(1):402. [PMC free article] [PubMed] [Google Scholar]

53. D'Agnelli S, Arendt-Nielsen L, Gerra MC, Zatorri K, Boggiani L, Baciarello M, Bignami E. Fibromyalgia: genetics and epigenetics insights may provide the basis for the development of diagnostic biomarkers. Mol Pain. 2019;15:1744806918819944. [PMC free article] [PubMed] [Google Scholar]

54. Corey DL, Comeau D. Cervical radiculopathy. Med Clin. 2014;98(4):791–799. [PubMed] [Google Scholar]
55. Woods BI, Hilibrand AS. Cervical radiculopathy. J Spinal Disord Tech. 2015;28(5):E251–E259. [PubMed] [Google Scholar]

56. McClune T, Burton AK, Waddell G. Whiplash associated disorders: a review of the literature to guide patient information and advice. Emerg Med J. 2002;19(6):499–506. [PMC free article] [PubMed] [Google Scholar]

57. Pastakia K, Kumar S. Acute whiplash associated disorders (WAD) Open Access Emerg Med. 2011;3:29. [PMC free article] [PubMed] [Google Scholar]

58. Poorbaugh K, Brismée JM, Phelps V, Sizer PS., Jr Late whiplash syndrome: a clinical science approach to evidence-based diagnosis and management. Pain Pract. 2008;8(1):65–89. [PubMed] [Google Scholar]

59. Gillick JL, Wainwright J, Das K. Rheumatoid arthritis and the cervical spine: a review on the role of surgery, Int J Rheumatol. 2015;2015:252456. [PMC free article] [PubMed]

60. Mańczak M, Gasik R. Cervical spine instability in the course of rheumatoid arthritis–imaging methods. Reumatologia. 2017;55(4):201. [PMC free article] [PubMed] [Google Scholar]

61. González-Gay MA, Matteson EL, Castañeda S. Polymyalgia rheumatica. Lancet. 2017;390(10103):1700–1712. [PubMed] [Google Scholar]

62. Guggino G, Ferrante A, Macaluso F, Triolo G, Ciccia F. Pathogenesis of polymyalgia rheumatica. Reumatismo. 2018;70(1):10–7. [PubMed]

63. O'Connor AB, Schwid SR, Herrmann DN, Markman JD, Dworkin RH. Late whiplash syndrome: a clinical science approach to evidence-based diagnosis and management. PAIN® 2008;137(1):96–111. [PubMed] [Google Scholar]

64. Ranganathan V, Gracey E, Brown MA, Inman RD, Haroon N. Pathogenesis of ankylosing spondylitis— recent advances and future directions. Nat Rev Rheumatol. 2017;13(6):359. [PubMed] [Google Scholar]

65. Bliddal H, Danneskiold-Samsøe B. Chronic widespread pain in the spectrum of rheumatological diseases. Best Pract Res Clin Rheumatol. 2007;21(3):391–402. [PubMed] [Google Scholar]

66. McGrath ER, Doughty CT, Amato AA. Autoimmune myopathies: updates on evaluation and treatment. Neurotherapeutics. 2018;15(4):976–994. [PMC free article] [PubMed] [Google Scholar]

67. Cantini F, Niccoli L, Nannini C, Kaloudi O, Bertoni M, Cassara E. Psoriatic arthritis: a systematic review. Int J Rheum Dis. 2010;13(4):300–317. [PubMed] [Google Scholar]

68. Fejer R, Hartvigsen J, Kyvik KO. Heritability of neck pain: a population-based study of 33 794 Danish twins. Rheumatology. 2006;45(5):589–594. [PubMed] [Google Scholar]

69. Hartvigsen J, Nielsen J, Kyvik KO, Fejer R, Vach W, Iachine I, Leboeuf-Yde C. Heritability of spinal pain and consequences of spinal pain: a comprehensive genetic epidemiologic analysis using a population-based sample of 15,328 twins ages 20–71 years. Arthritis Care Res. 2009;61(10):1343–1351. [PubMed] [Google Scholar]

70. MacGregor AJ, Andrew T, Sambrook PN, Spector TD. Structural, psychological, and genetic influences on low back and neck pain: a study of adult female twins. Arthritis Care Res. 2004;51(2):160–167. [PubMed] [Google Scholar]

71. Nyman T, Mulder M, Iliadou A, Svartengren M, Wiktorin C. High heritability for concurrent low back and neck-shoulder pain: a study of twins. Spine. 2011;36(22):E1469–E1476. [PubMed] [Google Scholar]

72. Ståhl MK, El-Metwally AA, Mikkelsson MK, Salminen JJ, Pulkkinen LR, Rose RJ, Kaprio JA. Genetic and environmental influences on non-specific neck pain in early adolescence: a classical twin study. Eur J Pain. 2013;17(6):791–798. [PMC free article] [PubMed] [Google Scholar]

73. Wang G, Cao Y, Wu T, Duan C, Wu J, Hu J, Lu H. Genetic factors of cervical spondylotic myelopathy-a systemic review. J Clin Neurosci. 2017;44:89–94. [PubMed] [Google Scholar]

74. Hartvigsen J, Pedersen HC, Frederiksen H, Christensen K. Small effect of genetic factors on neck pain in old age: a study of 2,108 Danish twins 70 years of age and older. Spine. 2005;30(2):206–208. [PubMed] [Google Scholar]

75. Meng W, Chan BW, Harris C, Freidin MB, Hebert HL, Adams MJ, Campbell A, Hayward C, Zheng H, Zhang X. A genome-wide association study finds genetic variants associated with neck or shoulder pain in UK biobank. Hum Mol Genet. 2020;29(8):1396–1404. [PMC free article] [PubMed] [Google Scholar]

76. Côté P, Cassidy JD, Carroll LJ, Kristman V. The annual incidence and course of neck pain in the general population: a population-based cohort study. Pain. 2004;112(3):267–273. [PubMed] [Google Scholar]

77. Jun D, Zoe M, Johnston V, O'Leary S. Physical risk factors for developing non-specific neck pain in office workers: a systematic review and meta-analysis. Int Arch Occup Environ Health. 2017;90(5):373–410. [PubMed] [Google Scholar]

78. Blyth FM, Huckel Schneider C. Global burden of pain and global pain policy—creating a purposeful body of evidence. PAIN. 2018;159(11):S43–8. [PubMed]

79. Cieza A, Causey K, Kamenov K, Hanson SW, Chatterji S, Vos T. Global estimates of the need for rehabilitation based on the global burden of disease study 2019: a systematic analysis for the global burden of disease study 2019. Lancet. 2020;396(10267):2006–2017. [PMC free article] [PubMed] [Google Scholar]

80. DALYs GBD, Collaborators H Global, regional, and national disability-adjusted life-years (DALYs) for 333 diseases and injuries and healthy life expectancy (HALE) for 195 countries and territories, 1990-2016: a systematic analysis for the global burden of disease study 2016. Lancet. 2017;390(10100):1260–1344. [PMC free article] [PubMed] [Google Scholar]

81. Miyamoto GC, Lin CC, Cabral CMN, van Dongen JM, van Tulder MW. Cost-effectiveness of exercise therapy in the treatment of non-specific neck pain and low back pain: a systematic review with meta-analysis. Br J Sports Med. 2019;53(3):172–181. [PubMed] [Google Scholar]

82. Fares J, Fares MY, Fares Y. Musculoskeletal neck pain in children and adolescents: risk factors and complications. Surg Neurol Int. 2017;8:72. [PMC free article] [PubMed] [Google Scholar]

83. Scarabottolo CC, Pinto RZ, Oliveira CB, Zanuto EF, Cardoso JR, Christofaro DGD. Back and neck pain prevalence and their association with physical inactivity domains in adolescents. Eur Spine J. 2017;26(9):2274–2280. [PubMed] [Google Scholar]

84. Minghelli B. Musculoskeletal spine pain in adolescents: epidemiology of non-specific neck and low back pain and risk factors. J Orthop Sci. 2020;25(5):776–780. [PubMed] [Google Scholar]

85. Croft PR, Lewis M, Papageorgiou AC, Thomas E, Jayson MIV, Macfarlane GJ, Silman AJ. Risk factors for neck pain: a longitudinal study in the general population. Pain. 2001;93(3):317–325. [PubMed] [Google Scholar]

www.ingramcontent.com/pod-product-compliance
Lightning Source LLC
Chambersburg PA
CBHW071714170526
45165CB00005B/2011